They Said Months.
I Chose Years!

J. R. O'Connor

Cancer Monthly, Inc.

They Said Months. I Chose Years!
A Mesothelioma Survivor's Story
J. R. O'Connor

Cancer Monthly, Inc.
14460 New Falls of Neuse Road, Suite 149-243
Raleigh, North Carolina 27614

Visit our websites:
http//www.cancermonthly.com
http//www.mycancerplace.com

Contact us:
info@cancermonthly.com

Cataloguing-in-Publication data
O'Connor, J.R.
They Said Months, I Chose Years: A Mesothelioma Survivor's
Story
Includes index.

ISBN 978-0-9772901-2-3

1. Cancer – Patients – Rehabilitation. 2. Mesothelioma –
Survival. 3. Cancer – Alternative therapies.

Cover Photo of J. R. O'Connor taken in 2008

10 9 8 7 6 5 4 3 2 1

ℬℭ

DEDICATION

I have written this book with the aspiration that it will give hope to those who are facing a cancer diagnosis and to enlighten them about other treatment approaches that may be of value.

I would like to take this opportunity to thank all of those without whose help I am sure that I would not have survived to write this book. My wife Arlene who is my caregiver and who makes sure that my daily regimen is faithfully followed and has supported me through out these years of trial with her unrelenting faith and perseverance in all things. My family and friends who have given their continuing prayers and support at all times in so very many ways. I especially want to thank my Nutritionist, Judith Todero and my Hypnotherapist, Dr. Don Morris who have given me guidance through these last few years.

And my thanks to our father in heaven every day. I have been fortunate to receive his many blessings and guidance through the years of my fight with this disease

$\text{\textbf{808}}$

DISCLAIMER

This book is based on the experiences of James O'Connor, a mesothelioma patient, and should be used for general information purposes only. None of this information in this book is a substitute for professional medical advice, examination, diagnosis or treatment and you should always seek the advice of your physician or other qualified health professional before starting any new treatment or making any changes to an existing treatment.

CONTENTS

$$\wp$$

INTRODUCTION

On October 15, 2001, I awoke from the anesthesia. I was lying in a bed in a hospital room at Kaiser Permanente Riverside Medical Center in Riverside, California. My wife, Arlene, and my two daughters sat at the end of the bed. I could tell that my thoracic surgeon had already talked to them because they appeared to be in a state of shock. I wondered what it meant.

I had just endured a chest biopsy in which tissue and fluid were removed from the pleural lining that covers my chest wall. Later I would find out that, as I slept, the surgeon had told my wife and daughters that he suspected that it was cancer and my life was in jeopardy, but a definitive diagnosis would have to wait the results of the pathologist's examination of the biopsy material.

"They think it may be some kind of cancer," my wife said gently.

I looked at her and said "Don't worry, I will be okay."

Perhaps it was the anesthesia or my drowsiness talking, but I really was not worried. Deep in my heart, I knew I would be okay and that I would survive.

Soon I was discharged and spent the next two weeks at home waiting the definitive diagnosis. I went on with my life focusing on the future as best I could. I went fishing and flew radio controlled airplanes, two of my favorite pastimes.

During this two week period there were times when I forgot that I was awaiting a verdict from the doctors. Then it would come crashing back in and I would remember what I was waiting for. During those moments my life felt like it was on hold until I heard the diagnosis and prognosis. But, then a voice somewhere in my mind said that it didn't matter. Whatever the doctors said, I knew I could conquer it.

Finally, two weeks came and went and I heard nothing so I drove to the hospital and spoke to a nurse. She told me that some, not all, of the biopsy samples had come back from the pathologist and that I would have to wait for the surgeon to return from vacation to hear what the findings were. Great, more suspense, I thought to myself.

About ten days later I went to the hospital for my follow-up appointment with the surgeon. It was time to take the staples out of my chest – the ones that were holding the skin in place over the biopsy sites. Casually, the doctor said that I had mesothelioma.

"Meso what?" I said.

"Mesothelioma," he repeated.

"What is that?" I asked.

"Mesothelioma. In your case it's cancer on the pleura. You will have to speak with the oncologist," the surgeon said matter of factly.

"It is definitely cancer?"

"Yes."

"How did I get it?" I asked.

"It comes from asbestos. The oncologist should be able to answer all your questions," he said.

I immediately attempted to make an appointment with the oncologist only to be told that the soonest appointment available would be in two weeks. Two more weeks to wait.

More suspense.

At this point all I had was a disease and a name. No real explanation, no treatment plan, no prognosis, no support, no answers. Just questions. Lots of them.

Two weeks later, I had my appointment with the medical oncologist. My wife and I sat together in a small examination room as he explained what mesothelioma was, that it was considered a "terminal" cancer, that I had less than a year to live, and that the various treatment options included chemotherapy, radiation, and surgery. In my case, he explained, surgery was not possible because, according to the surgeon, the surgical margins would require removing parts of my backbone – an unacceptable risk. Radiation was also not an option, he explained, because my cancer was so widespread it would mean radiating the entire chest cavity which would do more harm than good. Chemo was the only viable option and it might give me a few extra months to live but at a cost – it would severely and negatively impact my quality of life. Finally, he said there were also clinical trials of experimental therapies available for mesothelioma and that if I were interested I could go online to the National Cancer Institute website to see a list of them.

"What about alternative medicine?" I asked. "Vitamins, herbs, diet and those types of things?"

"Don't waste your money on the quacks," he said.

I was quiet. I was thinking. My wife said nothing.

The doctor added, "Spend your money wisely. Take Arlene on a nice cruise. When you come back we can set you up with hospice if you like."

The pessimism continued a few more minutes. It was clear that for this doctor my untimely death was preordained. Soon the consultation was over. Arlene appeared visibly shaken. I wasn't. While I was little surprised by the oncologist's crass bedside manner, I still wasn't worried. Before I had even walked into the oncologist's examination room I had already decided what I was going to do.

Approximately, seven months after this consultation, in June 2002, I would see the first evidence that my tumors were shrinking. The oncologist had insisted that I monitor the cancer with X-rays, but my research had revealed that X-rays lacked the precision to detect and measure subtle changes in mesothelioma. I insisted on a CT or CAT scan. Finally the doctor agreed. Comparing this CT against the CT taken at the time of my diagnosis revealed the change – the tumors were regressing. The doctor was amazed. Nine months after diagnosis, about the time I should be on my death-bed, I was actually getting better.

Since that day in June 2002, my mesothelioma has continued to regress. It is not gone. As I will explain in the chapters ahead, the goal of alternative medicine is not to eliminate a tumor, but rather to make sure that the tumor does not kill the patient. The approaches I used were, on the surface, simple. However, they required knowledge, commitment and discipline. This book explains them all.

In a nutshell, I took an approach based on self-reliance. As I outline in Chapter One, I was willing to challenge the precepts and assumptions of conventional medicine because it had little to offer me. As I describe in Chapters Two and Three, I focused on strengthening the body through diet, vitamins, and other supplements. This, in my opinion, is very important. In Chapters Four, Five and Six I present medical evidence that

4

lends support to the belief that alternative medicine can be of value to cancer patients. In Chapter Seven I also discuss mind-body medicine because I think this is an important approach also. Finally, in Chapter Eight, I talk about making treatment decisions.

I have also included seven appendices that I think are of value. Appendix 1 presents dietary reference intake values for vitamins and elements. Appendix 2 outlines some questions you may want to ask your doctors when learning about various treatment options. Appendix 3 is a reprint of an interview with Paul Kraus. Paul is a fellow mesothelioma victim who is alive eleven years after being diagnosed. Like me, he also used alternative approaches. Appendix 4 discusses the importance of getting the right pathology diagnosis. And Appendix 5 presents some ideas on how to conduct valid and reliable research on alternative therapies. Appendix 6 lists the alternative licensed clinicians I work with. And Appendix 7 lists additional articles about cancer and nutrition.

Of course, a book like this has to come with caveats. There is no guarantee whatsoever that what worked for me will work for others. Everyone must find their own path to healing whether it is with conventional treatments like surgery or chemotherapy, clinical trials, or alternative or integrative medicine. Also, I am not against conventional medicine. There is a role for every type of therapy. I believe, however, when conventional medicine has nothing or little to offer that it makes sense to look at other treatment options that may be available.

My wish and prayer for all who read my book is that it will strengthen and inspire you to do whatever it takes to not only survive your disease, but also to thrive and enjoy your life.

ಛ 1 ೞ

SELF SUFFICIENCY

IS IT POSSIBLE TO MANAGE A DISEASE LIKE CANCER USING NON-CONVENTIONAL MEANS? In my opinion the answer is a resounding yes! But, that does not mean that there is a magic bullet in the form of a specific herb or vitamin. I wish there was, but I don't think there is. At least I have not found it. It also does not mean that there isn't a role for conventional treatments. Heck, when chemo is a cure I will be the first to sign-up. The problem is that most times, especially with mesothelioma and other advanced solid cancers, it is not. In fact, choosing an alternative approach is more complicated than chemotherapy, radiation or surgery because with the holistic modalities there is no "one size fits all."

For example, if you have mesothelioma the chemotherapy regimen today is a combination of two drugs – pemetrexed (Alimta) and cisplatin or carboplatin. Typically, your age, cell type and staging will not dictate the kind of chemo you receive as first-line treatment. If your doctors recommend chemo, chances are that Alimta plus a platinum drug will be prescribed.

With alternative modalities, however, there are many different approaches. These approaches are based (or should be based) on the specific needs of the patient. Because all patients are individuals and their needs are all individualistic you can imagine that these therapies can take many forms. What works for me will probably not work for anyone else because what is going on in my body is probably different than what is going on

6

in yours. That is why it is important to work with professional clinicians if you decide to go down the alternative road. A professional trained in this area is needed to figure out what exactly you need.

Now, here's another fact to consider – a naturopathic doctor or nutritionist cannot treat cancer. It is against the law. It fact, in some states, chemo, radiation and surgery are the only legal therapies for cancer. How then can a clinician treat cancer using non-traditional means? The answer is that they can't!

This is a critical point that is important to understand. While a medical oncologist treats cancer, a clinician using alternative approaches does not. The alternative clinician can only suggest various herbs, vitamins, and other natural modalities designed to give the patient's body what the body needs to manage the cancer. In other words, with a medical oncologist or surgeon the intervention itself (chemo or surgery) is designed to directly impact the cancer. In contract, alternative practitioners never treat the cancer, but treat the patient instead. The concept is that once the patient is strengthened or given what is missing then the patient's body can manage the cancer itself through its immune system and other biological processes. This explains why alternative practitioners don't talk about cancer treatment or cancer cures. They can't. Plus, this is not what they do. They treat the patient.

Also, when conventional doctors talk about how alternative approaches are unproven they are essentially correct. If by "proven" they mean that there have been clinical studies that have demonstrated a survival advantage with alternative approaches. In fact, while there have been thousands of studies that have demonstrated that certain herbs, vitamins, and mushrooms can kill various cancers in test tubes there have been very few studies that have tested them in actual patients. Let's think about this for a second. There are many studies that demonstrate that these natural approaches kill cancer *in vitro* (in test tubes and Petrie dishes) yet the studies never went any further. They were never tested in patients. Why is this? The answer is economic.

The Economics of Cancer Treatments

The Food and Drug Administration (FDA) does not allow all potential cancer treatments to reach the market, only those that they approve after a drug company invests an estimated $500 million to take the treatment through clinical trials. Drug companies, however, will only invest that much money in treatments they can patent. A patent allows the pharmaceutical company to control the product, set the price, and make as much profit as possible. The problem, of course, is that patentable cancer drugs are by definition synthetic; they are made in a lab. This shuts out virtually every naturally occurring compound that already exists in nature and explains why no mushroom, vitamin, herb, or other naturally occurring whole entity has ever been FDA approved for the treatment of cancer.

This makes it tough on the cancer patient. The patient must first understand that alternative approaches address the patient, not the cancer. In a culture where we see TV commercials for specific drugs designed to directly treat specific ailments this principle is challenging to accept.

Next, patients have to acknowledge the truth of what their conventional doctors tell them – that nearly all alternative approaches are unproven in the treatment of cancer. Of course, what is left out is the fact that they are unproven because no one has paid to do the testing in patients. What is also left out is that there are countless anecdotal reports of cancer patients given up for dead by conventional doctors who used alternative modalities to return them to health. And what is also left out is that there are many compelling studies in animals and human cancer cell lines that have demonstrated that various naturally occurring substances can kill or arrest cancer.

Third, it can be very difficult to find an experienced, educated, well trained alternative clinician who can work with a cancer patient to help restore them to health. (Notice again that I did not say remove or cure the cancer because they don't do this.)

Is there a solution to these challenges? I think everyone has to find their own path when facing a terminal disease. The patient should listen to and weigh the advice of their conventional doctors. If there is no cure or there may be a cure but at a terrible price of quality of life then I think it make sense to explore other options. After all it is your life, not the doctor's. That is where self reliance and self sufficiency come in. Without an inner faith in yourself and your own decisions it can be almost impossible to keep an open mind and challenge convention.

Self Sufficiency

How important is self-sufficiency in surviving mesothelioma or any other cancer? I think it is vital. You have to possess the faith and confidence to make the right treatment decisions. Many patients spend hours, days or weeks second-guessing themselves about what they would have or could have or should have done. This is very unproductive.

Focus on Today

There is always a tomorrow, but never a yesterday. You cannot change the past, but you can always use what you learned in the past to make better decisions now.

I have never been a person who worries about things. As a young man, when I was discharged from of the Marine Corps, I married Arlene and she already had three children. Now here I was with not much of a resume or money and I already had four mouths to feed plus myself. I imagine other men in my position would have questioned and doubted themselves and their decisions. I didn't. I knew that I loved Arlene. I also knew that whatever happens happens and you cannot go through life second guessing yourself because that is not living.

How can you make the most of the present if you are dreading what you did in the past? As it turned out, our family life was wonderful. Of course there were bumps in the road like everyone else and plenty of financial ups and downs, but we lived our lives together and I never wasted time or energy trying to change the unchangeable past.

Perform Your Research and Keep an Open Mind

But there is more to self sufficiency than minimizing self-doubt. No matter how confident you are, if you have no information or the wrong information you will make poor decisions. This goes for cancer or anything else. There is an old computer term "GIGO" which stands for "garbage in, garbage out." If you fill your mind with accurate, fact based information then your decisions, based on that information, will be accurate and fact based. But, if you fill your mind with inaccurate information and garbage then that's what you will get – bad decisions! This is especially true for making cancer treatment decisions.

On October 15, 2001 I had my biopsy and learned that I probably had mesothelioma, but it wasn't until six weeks later that I learned about the treatment options offered by the oncologist.

I spent much of that month and a half learning all I could about the disease. I read about the treatment options and discovered how they were generally ineffective in most mesothelioma patients. I also found out that chemotherapy and the more drastic surgeries that are commonly used, and radiation to a lesser extent, all significantly and negatively impacted ones quality of life. I had a pretty good quality of life at the moment and I wanted to sustain it. It just did not make sense to me to make myself sick in order to get well.

So, I decided to keep an open mind and read about alternative therapies and discovered that they were modeled on Eastern philosophies and medicine. For example, the goal of Eastern medicine is to treat diseases by removing their cause. In contrast the goal of Western medicine is to treat diseases by removing their symptoms. In cancer, Western medicine uses surgery, chemotherapy or radiation to, respectively, cut, poison or burn the tumor. But what actually *caused* the tumor in mesothelioma or any cancer? Western medicine believes that the tumor is both the symptom of the disease and also the disease itself. This did not make sense to me.

Consider other diseases like diabetes, heart disease or scurvy. In type II diabetes, the symptoms include a raised glucose level. But a raised glucose level is not the disease. The disease is' actually caused by not producing enough insulin or the cells ignoring the insulin.

In heart disease, the symptoms include angina or chest pain, shortness of breath, and palpitations. Are these the causes of the disease? No, the causes can be too much bad cholesterol, obesity, tobacco use, or a number of other issues.

In scurvy, the patient's teeth fall out. Is the fallen tooth the disease or just a manifestation of the disease? Obviously it's just a symptom. The cause is a lack of vitamin C.

As I learned more, I realized that I did not buy-in to the Western philosophy that a tumor is both the symptom and the cause of cancer. If it were, then early diagnosis and wide excisions (surgeries with wide margins that remove all the cancer) should always result in a cure. But they did not.

But, there were even other reasons why the Western philosophy didn't make sense to me. A big one was asbestos.

Asbestos and Mesothelioma

Asbestos is a naturally occurring mineral that is known to cause mesothelioma. This mineral has been used in thousands of products and applications. Now, I had worked around asbestos and had been exposed to this carcinogen. But, so had my co-workers and the overwhelming majority of them were not diagnosed with mesothelioma or any other cancer. They probably had asbestos fibers in their body, like I did, but these carcinogenic fibers never created cancer in them. Why I wondered.

In addition, mesothelioma has a long latency period – the time from asbestos exposure to actually getting the disease. This latency period could range from 20 years to more than 50 years.

This means that I, like other patients with this disease, had asbestos in my body for decades before it caused me any trouble.

I felt that these two questions were important. If asbestos causes mesothelioma, which it does, how come most people exposed to this carcinogen never get the disease? Second, why do those individuals who get the disease have a latency period of many decades? For me the obvious answer was that there was something else going on within the bodies of people that allowed the cancer to erupt after so many years. I wondered what else could it be?

The Immune System and Cancer

I continued my research and read about the immune system and how there are specific cells in our body such as "natural killer cells" that function to eliminate cancer cells. I read how some doctors believed that everyone has cancer cells forming all the time and the immune system is equipped to eliminate them so that they do not cause disease.

In fact, a leading medical text book stated that the immune system can recognize and eliminate malignant tumors. According to Harrison's Principles of Internal Medicine, "Animal studies have conclusively shown that the immune system can recognize and eliminate malignant tumors in vivo (in the body)."[1]

And according to the National Cancer Institute website: "According to one theory, patrolling cells of the immune system provide continuous body wide surveillance, catching and eliminating cells that undergo malignant transformation. Tumors develop when this immune surveillance breaks down or is overwhelmed."[2]

---

[1] Harrison's Principles of Internal Medicine, 14th Edition, Biologic Therapy, p. 535.

[2] National Cancer Institute – Understanding Cancer Series: The Immune System. Available here:
http://www.cancer.gov/cancertopics/understandingcancer/
immunesystem/allpages

This made sense to me because it helped answer those two basic questions: If asbestos causes cancer how come most people exposed to this carcinogen never get the disease and why do those people who get the disease have a latency period of many decades? Perhaps if "tumors develop when this immune surveillance breaks down or is overwhelmed" then the disease erupts with the breakdown of the immune system. This does not mean that asbestos doesn't cause mesothelioma. It most certainly does. Study after study has demonstrated this. But, a breakdown of the immune system may be the final straw that leads to disease in people exposed to this carcinogen. In fact, maybe a healthy immune system is able to keep the asbestos fibers in check and stop them from causing tumors. If this assumption was true, and I realized it was just my assumption, it would mean that my immune system and its malfunctioning contributed to my mesothelioma diagnosis and the tumors were just the result of this underlying problem. So I wondered what could overwhelm my immune system?

Protecting the Immune System

According to the prestigious Cleveland Clinic[3], the three areas that are most important in protecting and bolstering the immune system are:

1. Diet and Nutrition;
2. Exercise;
3. Stress Reduction.

I realized that I had neglected all three in recent years.

---

[3] Diet, Exercise, Stress, and the Immune System, Cleveland Clinic Center for Consumer Health Information available at: http://www.clevelandclinic.org/health/health-info/docs/0900/0955.asp?index=5429

Diet and Nutrition

Up until the time of my mesothelioma diagnosis, my diet had been pretty poor. I ate a lot of meat. Hamburgers were one of my favorites. And I ate lots of fried foods too. According to the Cleveland Clinic a healthy immune system depended in part on a diet with sufficient antioxidants and enough nutrients and micronutrients. This I needed to address.

Exercise

Also, according to the Cleveland Clinic, "Even more so than nutrition, exercise has the capacity to protect and even enhance the immune response. Experimental studies have shown that a regular exercise program of brisk walking can bolster many defenses of the immune system, including the antibody response and the natural killer (T cell) response."[4]

Prior to my diagnosis, my exercise regimen had been pretty non-existent. In fact I had no exercise regimen. Although I played golf two or three times a week and enjoyed flying my radio controlled airplanes, I did nothing that required me to break a sweat.

Stress

In addition, many scientists believe that chronic stress can suppress one's immune system. For example, according to Dr. Esther Sternberg, director of the Integrative Neural Immune Program at the National Institute of Health's National Institute of Mental Health (NIMH), "if you're chronically stressed, the part of the brain that controls the stress response is going to be constantly pumping out a lot of stress hormones. The immune

---

[4] Diet, Exercise, Stress, and the Immune System, Cleveland Clinic Center for Consumer Health Information available at:
http://www.clevelandclinic.org/health/health-info/docs/0900/0955.asp?index=5429

cells are being bathed in molecules which are essentially telling them to stop fighting. And so in situations of chronic stress your immune cells are less able to respond to an invader like a bacteria or a virus."[5]

In fact, prior to my diagnosis I had gone through a period of extensive stress. I owned and operated a dry cleaning plant and two dry cleaning stores. The hours were long and the work was tiring. There was always plenty to do and much to worry about.

Process of Finding Your Healing Path

From everything I had read, I decided that an alternative healing approach that addressed what I believed to be my underlying problems of lack of immune competence was best suited for me. What I have come to learn since that decision seven years ago, is that this was the correct decision in my case. But, I have also learned a bigger lesson that cancer patients can benefit from going through a process of finding their own healing path. What worked for me may not work for others and what worked for others may not work for me. What is important, however, is the process of questioning, researching, and discovering. These steps can eventually lead to a patient embracing the best healing modalities for them.

For example, there are some patients that just do what the doctors tell them and don't believe in the treatment at all. I am not against listening to doctors. My point, however, is that if someone is embarking on a treatment for which they have no belief and no faith then there is a problem. If you agree on a therapy because your doctor recommended it and deep in your soul it feels right – this is powerful. But, if your heart you have strong doubts about the treatment then your mind and body may be trying to tell you something.

---

[5] Stress and Disease: New Perspectives, The NIH Word on Health
By Harrison Wein, Ph.D. available at:
http://www.nih.gov/news/WordonHealth/oct2000/story01.htm

Writers like Bernie Siegel, M.D. have observed that cancer patients who survive longer and have a better quality of life have four faiths: faith in oneself, one's doctor, one's treatment and one's spiritual faith. If you don't believe in your treatment, no matter how good it is, you may be setting yourself up for failure.

By the time I started my alternative therapies I knew that whether I lived or died this was the therapy destined for me. Out of this belief I had total confidence in the healing path I had chosen. This was powerful.

The Importance of a Caregiver

Another source of self sufficiency and confidence came from the total support from my own personal caregiver, Arlene, my wife. You can be a self confident person like I was and take the steps necessary to embrace the treatment that feels right for you, but if you are totally alone it is still a difficult road. Arlene was there every step of the way. She accompanied me to doctor visits, asked questions, and supported my decisions.

According to the American Academy of Family Physicians, asking your family members for help when you are diagnosed with cancer benefits you and them. According to their website, "Members of your family want to give you their support, but aren't always sure how. Assign specific tasks to each individual. If one person in your family is particularly organized, ask him or her to help you handle insurance and legal issues. Have a family member collect and write down any questions that you and your family have for your doctor. Take this person with you when you visit your doctor. Your family member can make sure all of the questions are asked and record the answers."[6]

---

[6] Cancer: Helping Your Family Help You from The American Academy of Family Physicians available at:
http://familydoctor.org/online/famdocen/home/common/cancer/treatment/728.html

Arlene and I did this instinctively and this helped me immensely because I did not have to face this cancer challenge alone. I was part of a team.

You Have to Be Disciplined

I believe that discipline has helped me survive my diagnosis. In fact, I probably wouldn't be here without it. Discipline or self-discipline provides the stamina to persevere. It bestows the ability to withstand hardships and difficulties, whether physical, emotional or mental. It grants the ability to reject immediate satisfaction for something better. Turning away from conventional therapies and embarking on my own path to treat my disease took discipline and courage.

I don't want to give the wrong impression. Of course I had doubts and second thoughts. But once I made my decision as to my treatment course of choice, I challenged myself to maintain focus and discipline in order to see it through.

When I was younger I was quite athletic and played football, basketball, and baseball. I even went to college on a football scholarship. Playing sports, I learned that you have to ignore the little things, stay focused and committed to the bigger goal, push forward and play through pain.

Now, I exercise discipline every day. Many times I don't feel like exercising, but I do it. Sometimes I don't want to eat my healthy diet, but I do it. Some days I don't want to take the hundred supplement pills that I am supposed to take every day, but I do it. For me it's all about discipline.

Believe in Something Greater Than Yourself

As a Mormon, I have a strong religious background. I believe in something greater than myself. I also believe that I am being helped. Having this belief has given me strength. I am not suggesting that religious belief per se is necessary, rather a belief in something outside yourself can be an important source of strength and inspiration. Whatever your beliefs, I think you

17

will agree that a Creator would not put us on this earth to suffer and die prematurely, but would want us to survive and thrive. If you think about that and realize that there is a life force that wants you to continue to live then you realize that your destiny is with the living.

As you no doubt see that what I am calling "self sufficiency" actually does require help from others. However, it is the kind of help that does not weaken and cause dependency, but strengthens your resolve to find, embrace and realize your own path to health and healing.

ഔ 2 ର

DIET & HEALTH

I BELIEVE THAT DIET, WHAT YOU PUT IN YOUR BODY, IS THE KEY TO HEALTH. To use an obvious analogy, if you put bad gas into your car would you expect it to run well? Of course not. Higher octane fuel gives your car better performance. It's the same thing with the human body. If you put premium "high octane" products into your body, you can expect better performance.

Our diets can effect us immediately and also over a longer-term. For example, what I eat today may be burned for energy tomorrow. And some of the raw ingredients that keep us healthy have to be ingested continually because we cannot manufacture them ourselves from the foods we eat. Other necessary dietary elements can actually be stored by our bodies. Therefore, what is running our body today may be the result of what we have eaten over several months. But, this picture becomes more complex if we consider the toxicities that may keep us from absorbing the nutrition we need and may actually keep our immune systems distracted.

Detoxification

Detoxification is a subject that is taken very seriously by many holistic and alternative practitioners. Max Gerson, M.D., an alternative physician who reportedly treated cancer successfully using detoxification and nutrition was one of the

19

first to write about the subject. Of course, nearly all conventional cancer doctors believe that our body's state of toxicity (or lack of toxicity) have absolutely no bearing on our cancer diagnosis or prognosis. I disagree. I believe that there are so many toxic chemicals in our food, water, and air that they can accumulate in our organs. If these toxic accumulations negatively impact the organ's functioning then the body pays a price.

During my first visit with my nutritionist, she told me that we needed to clean out my system. She explained that if my liver and kidneys were clean and less toxic then they would filter the blood appropriately and the blood (including the white blood cells that are inside) could then function more optimally. She explained that the same applied to my colon and digestive tract. She said that if they were clean and functioning optimally then the nutritional foods and supplements that I ingested could be more fully utilized and I would receive the maximum benefit.

In addition to filtering and cleaning my blood more efficiently, I learned that detoxification could potentially benefit my immune system in another way. Toxins such as chemicals, artificial hormones, heavy metals, pesticides, herbicides and fungicides in our food and water may stay in the colon for many years. In fact, I have read that the Environmental Protection Agency (EPA) estimates that nearly a half a million different chemicals are used today, and that 5,000 new chemical substances are added each year. Once inside the body, these unhealthy, exogenous substances may trigger the immune system. After all, the immune system is designed to attack and eliminate foreign invaders. If the immune system becomes distracted by fighting toxic foreign invaders, how much of this system is left to fight serious diseases like cancer?

To help in my detoxification process, I used a variety of products and supplements under the care of my nutritionist. These included: Natures Life Ultimate Fiber and Ultimate Herbs (after a couple of years I changed to the Super Cleanse), lecithin, thisilin, and marshmallow (the herb not the confection).

My Diet

Since my mesothelioma diagnosis I have been working with my nutritionist who helps me manage my diet and supplements. My diet consists of range-fed beef (about once a week) and no other red or white meats. I especially stay away from any animal protein that contains added hormones. In some cancers, the cancer cells can have hormone receptors and artificial or supplemental hormones can trigger these cells to multiply. I also eat a lot of fresh fish and vegetables. I try to make sure these foods are wholesome and organically grown if possible. In addition, I have cut out all sugar, hydrogenated oils, and fried foods.

I focus on organic foods and try to stay away from foods that are sprayed with chemicals. For example, most stores will spray fruits and vegetables (even those that are organic) with water that contains chemicals to enhance their color. Therefore, we always wash produce with a light vinegar solution to eliminate the toxins so we do not ingest them.

No Sugar

I have read that the average American consumes between two and three pounds of sugar each week. That's an incredible statistic! Highly refined sugars come in a variety of forms including: sucrose (table sugar), dextrose (corn sugar), and high-fructose corn syrup. These forms can be found in many foods including bread, breakfast cereal, mayonnaise, peanut butter, and ketchup.

Sugar may act as fuel for cancer cell. Otto Warburg, Ph.D., the 1931 Nobel laureate in medicine, discovered that cancer cells have a fundamentally different energy metabolism compared to healthy cells. His Nobel thesis discussed the fact that malignant tumors frequently exhibit an increase in "anaerobic glycolysis" - a process whereby glucose is used by cancer cells as a fuel with lactic acid as an anaerobic by-product. Assuming this is correct,

21

the less glucose available, the less fuel there may be for cancer cells.

Sugar has also been recognized as raising the risk of certain cancers. For example, here is what some doctors and scientists have stated in their peer reviewed medical journals:

- "High consumption of sugar and high-sugar foods may be associated with a greater risk of pancreatic cancer."[7]

- "High intakes of dietary glycemic load, fructose, and sucrose were related to an elevated colorectal cancer risk among men."[8]

- "The study suggests that high sucrose intake could be an important risk factor in lung carcinogenesis."[9]

- "These findings support previous reports that dietary sugars, especially diet high in simple carbohydrates relative to complex carbohydrates, increase risk of colon cancer, possibly through their impact on plasma glucose levels."[10]

---

[7] Larsson SC, et al., Consumption of sugar and sugar-sweetened foods and the risk of pancreatic cancer in a prospective study. Am J Clin Nutr. 2006 Nov;84(5):1171-6.

[8] Michaud DS, et al., Dietary glycemic load, carbohydrate, sugar, and colorectal cancer risk in men and women. Cancer Epidemiol Biomarkers Prev. 2005 Jan;14(1):138-47.

[9] De Stefani E, et al., Dietary sugar and lung cancer: a case-control study in Uruguay. Nutr Cancer. 1998;31(2):132-7.

[10] Slattery ML, et al., Dietary sugar and colon cancer. Cancer Epidemiol Biomarkers Prev. 1997 Sep;6(9):677-85.

- "In older women a strong correlation was found between breast cancer mortality and sugar consumption…"[11]

Since sugar is devoid of minerals, vitamins, and fiber, has a negative effect on health and may fuel or increase one's risk for cancer, I have simply removed it from my diet as much as possible and I try to stay away from any foods that contain it.

No Hydrogenated Oils & Fried Foods

I also try to stay away from hydrogenated oils and fried foods because many fried foods contain these dangerous oils.

To increase their shelf life, certain oils are hydrogenated. This process turns the oil into a solid at room temperature, but it also makes the oil unhealthy by creating something called "trans fatty acids." Trans fatty acids increase total cholesterol levels and LDL cholesterol levels (the "bad" cholesterol), and reduce HDL cholesterol (the "good" cholesterol). The more solid the oil, the more the trans fatty acids inside. High-fat baked goods (especially doughnuts, cookies and cakes) and any product for which the label says "partially hydrogenated vegetable oils" (which includes almost all processed foods) contain trans fatty acids. While there doesn't seem to be any consensus on whether these hydrogenated oils and trans fatty acids can cause or contribute to cancer, there are some studies that may be early warnings. For example, here are some quotes from some recent scientific studies:

- "The trans fatty acids in partially hydrogenated vegetable oil may cause colorectal neoplasia by interfering with cell membrane function or eicosanoid metabolism."[12]

---

[11] Seely S, Horrobin DF. Diet and breast cancer: the possible connection with sugar consumption. Med Hypotheses. 1983 Jul;11(3):319-27.

- "There are multiple adverse effects of trans fatty acids (TFA) that are produced by partial hydrogenation (i.e., manufactured TFA), on CVD, blood lipids, inflammation, oxidative stress, endothelial health, body weight, insulin sensitivity, and cancer."[13]

- "Among Caucasians, we observed that each type of trans-fatty acid and total trans-fatty acid intake showed a statistically significant positive association with prostate cancer..."[14]

Why take the risk and consume products that contain these substances that are recognized as unhealthy? I try not to and that's why I avoid fried foods, snack foods, margarine, donuts, cakes, and other food products that may contain these trans fatty acids.

Yes to Good Fats & Oils

On the subject of oils, there are some that are very important for health. Contrary to popular belief, our bodies do need some of the right kinds of fats. Essential Fatty Acids (EFA's) are necessary to health and cannot be made by the body. (That's why they are called "essential.")

EFA's support the cardiovascular, reproductive, immune, and nervous systems. Every living cell in our bodies needs EFA's.

---

[12] McKelvey W, et al., A second look at the relation between colorectal adenomas and consumption of foods containing partially hydrogenated oils. Epidemiology. 2000 Jul;11(4):469-73.

[13] Gebauer SK, et al., The diversity of health effects of individual trans fatty acid isomers. Lipids. 2007 Sep;42(9):787-99.

[14] Liu X, Schumacher FR, et al., Trans-fatty acid intake and increased risk of advanced prostate cancer: modification by RNASEL R462Q variant. Carcinogenesis. 2007 Jun;28(6):1232-6.

Cells use it to repair cell membranes, obtain optimum nutrition, expel harmful waste products, and make new cells. In addition, a primary function of EFA's is the production of prostaglandins which are chemical messengers that regulate body functions such as heart rate, blood pressure, blood clotting, fertility, conception, and immunity.

There are two basic categories of EFA's: omega-3 and omega-6. Omega-3 includes alpha-linolenic acid and eicosapentaenoic acid. Omega-6 includes linoleic and gamma-linolenic acids. Flaxseeds and flaxseed oil are rich in omega-3 EFA's. In 1951, Dr. Johanna Budwig, a German biochemist and expert on fats and oils proposed a flaxseed oil diet. She is best known for suggesting the benefits of a combination of flax seed oil and cottage cheese in cancer. In fact, I take 3,000 mg of flaxseed oil every day.

ഔ 3 ര

MY SUPPLEMENTS

MY SUPPLEMENT REGIMEN EVOLVED OVER TIME. At one point I was taking 142 pills a day. Today I am down to around 100 daily. My vitamin bill is about $1,000 a month.

I do not consume all the supplements in one sitting. It makes it difficult for the body to assimilate so many things at once. In addition, consuming vitamins throughout the day enables my body to maintain more consistent levels of each supplement in the bloodstream. Therefore, I split up the various vitamins and dosages and take vitamins about eight times every day.

I have reprinted my supplement list below so remember the caveat that we discussed before – There is no guarantee whatsoever that what worked for me will work for others. Everyone must find their own path to healing. If you are interested in an alternative regime the best thing to do is to work with a professional clinician who can guide you appropriately. <u>Don't do what I do, talk to your doctor!</u>

My supplements can be divided into various categories including:

- Vitamins
- Minerals
- Vegetables and vegetable products
- Fruit and fruit products
- Oils

- Amino acids
- Enzymes and co-enzymes
- Herbs

The entire list is:

<u>Once per day</u>

Artichoke supplement
Grapefruit Pectin 500 mg
Alive Multi Vitamin
B-12 5,000 mcg
B-6 200 mg
Potassium   750 mg

<u>Twice per day</u>

Grape seed with resveratrol
Beta glucan
Coq10 120mg
Tocotrienols
Phosphatidylserine.   100 mg
Alpha Lipolic Acid   250 mg
Folic acid   800 mcg
Vitamin A 25,000 iu
Liver Vitality
Acidophilus 1000 mg
B complex
Fenu-Thyme 450 mg
Lycopene 20 mg
Raw Adrenal Tabs
Calcium-magnesium supplement – 500 mg calcium and 250 mg magnesium
Maitake Mushroom (liquid) I take 1/2 eye dropper twice a day when I feel that my mesothelioma may be recurring.

Three times per day

Vitamin C 2 grams 3 times a day and additional 2 grams one time a day for a total of 8 grams a day (plus an additional gram from my multivitamin)
Flaxseed oil 1000 mg
Vitamin B-1 100 mg + 150 mg in complex formula
All-Zyme double strength
Vitamin E 400 mg
L-Glutathione 100 mg
Pycnogenol 100mg
NAC

AM & PM

Essiac Tea — two ounces first thing in the morning and two just prior to bed or two ounces twice a day, one first thing in the morning and one just prior to bed.
Super Cleanse (1 pm 3 am)
Solaray Stress AM-PM

Others

AG-immune 6/day
NK-Immune 2/day
Yew tea – I drink a few cups a day when I feel my mesothelioma may be recurring.

All of these supplements could also be divided into two major categories – whole food products, and natural ingredients.

Whole food products like flaxseed oil, artichoke, and grapeseed are made from the whole food. The actual food may be concentrated or dehydrated, but it is intact. All of the chemistry within the food still exists. It may contain many different types of substances.

In contrast, what I am calling natural ingredients are just parts of a natural occurring food source. For example, you seldom

28

(perhaps never) find individual amino acids or vitamins as separate entities in nature. They are always part of something greater and more complex.

In my non-scientific opinion it makes sense to get as many of your supplements in the whole food form as possible. I believe that there may be added benefits. For example, there may be ingredients in the whole form that are important to health that we may not even know exist because they have not yet been identified. In addition, some of the ingredients in the whole food may be more beneficial because complimentary or synergistic ingredients may also be present.

What follows is a basic overview of <u>some</u> of the various supplements I have taken and continue to take. I have included a small amount of information on what each one is or does, what the Dietary Reference Intake is, and the dose I consume.

The Dietary Reference Intake is a system of nutrition recommendations from the Institute of Medicine. The measures I will be using are: 1) Recommended Dietary Allowances (RDA) which is the daily dietary intake level of a nutrient considered sufficient to meet the requirements of nearly all healthy individuals in each life-stage and gender group; and 2) Adequate Intake (AI) which is the amount believed to be adequate when no RDA has been established. Dietary Reference Intake Tables for most vitamins and elements is available in the Appendix.

Important Caveat – Reminder!

Everyone is an individual and therefore everybody's nutritional and vitamin needs are specific to that individual. Your supplement needs, dosages and frequencies must be tailored to you! Work with a professional clinician or nutritionist to find out what is right for you. Many of these supplements can actually be dangerous if taken in too high amounts. As you will read, I am taking very high doses of a number of supplements but, I am doing this under the advice and watchful eyes of professional clinicians.

If you are interested in taking supplements in excess of the U.S. Government's Dietary Reference Intakes or Recommended Dietary Allowances be sure to work with your doctor!

Vitamins

Vitamins are necessary for life. Without the proper vitamins in the proper amounts, our bodies could not perform the thousands of biochemical reactions that make life possible.

For humans there are 13 vitamins: 4 fat-soluble (A, D, E and K) and 9 water-soluble (8 B vitamins and vitamin C). For the most part, vitamins are obtained with food, but a few are obtained by other means. For example, microorganisms like certain beneficial bacteria in the intestine known as "gut flora" produce vitamin K and biotin, while one form of vitamin D is synthesized in the skin with the help of natural ultraviolet rays in sunlight. In addition, we can produce some vitamins from precursors that we consume in our diet. For example, vitamin A can be produced from beta carotene, and niacin can be produced from the amino acid tryptophan. Both beta carotene and tryptophan can be found in various foods.

Conventional medicine has known for some time that certain vitamin deficiencies lead to specific diseases. For example, a deficiency in vitamin C can lead to scurvy and a deficiency in vitamin D can lead to rickets. Many health authorities, however, are beginning to realize that vitamins may also be needed to ward off chronic diseases like cancer. Many of these authorities are coming around to the idea that some supplements can be a good idea. For example, according to the Harvard School of Public Health Website:

Multivitamins may lower your risk of cancer, heart disease, osteoporosis, and birth defects. That's a lot of bang for your *buck, literally. For as little as $10 a year, multivitamins are the cheapest health insurance you can buy.*[15]

Vitamin A

Vitamin A is a very important vitamin to maintaining health because it has many essential functions in the human body. According to the National Institute of Health:

Vitamin A is a group of compounds that play an important role in vision, bone growth, reproduction, cell division, and cell differentiation (in which a cell becomes part of the brain, muscle, lungs, blood, or other specialized tissue). Vitamin A helps regulate the immune system, which helps prevent or fight off infections by making white blood cells that destroy harmful bacteria and viruses. Vitamin A also may help lymphocytes (a type of white blood cell) fight infections more effectively. Vitamin A promotes healthy surface linings of the eyes and the respiratory, urinary, and intestinal tracts. When those linings break down, it becomes easier for bacteria to enter the body and cause infection. Vitamin A also helps the skin and mucous membranes function as a barrier to bacteria and viruses.[16]

There are a variety of forms of vitamin A and each has a slightly different name so it can be confusing to understand how they are related. In general, there are two categories of vitamin A, depending on whether the food source is an animal or a plant.

---

[15] Harvard School of Public Health – Multivitamins: A Quick Fix
Available at: http://www.hsph.harvard.edu/cancer/risk/multivitamins/basics/mulitvitamin_bet.htm

[16] Dietary Supplement Fact Sheet: Vitamin A and Carotenoids : Office of Dietary Supplements • National Institutes of Health. Available at: http://ods.od.nih.gov/factsheets/vitamina.asp

Animal Sources

Vitamin A found in foods that come from animals (such as liver and whole milk) is called "preformed vitamin A." It is absorbed in the form of retinol and the body can convert retinol into retinal and retinoic acid.

Plant Sources

Vitamin A that is found in colorful fruits and vegetables is called provitamin A carotenoid which can be converted into retinol by the body. Common provitamin A carotenoids from plants include: beta carotene, alpha-carotene, and beta-cryptoxanthin. Among these, beta-carotene is most efficiently made into retinol. Retinoic acid is currently used to treat different types of cancer. For example, a standard therapy for acute promyelocic leukemia is all-trans retinoic acid (a type of retinoic acid). According to an article published in a leading medical journal:

"At the cellular level, the anti-leukemia and anti-cancer activity of retinoids is the result of three main actions, cell-differentiation, growth inhibition and apoptosis."[17]

I take 50,000 international units (IU) of vitamin A each day plus an additional 15,000 international units that I receive in my multi-vitamin (such as beta carotene and gamma carotene). The recommended dietary allowance (RDA) is 900 micrograms a day for men and 700 micrograms for women. So I take quite a bit more. But, remember the RDA recommends the average daily dietary intake level that is sufficient to meet the nutrient requirements of healthy individuals. Because I am dealing with a chronic disease – cancer, I don't consider myself in that group.

---

[17] Garattini E, et al., Retinoids as differentiating agents in oncology: a network of interactions with intracellular pathways as the basis for rational therapeutic combinations. Curr Pharm Des. 2007;13(13):1375-400.

Nonetheless, as the caveat at the beginning of this chapter states, everyone is an individual and therefore everybody's nutritional and vitamin needs are specific to that individual. Don't take what I am taking. Work with a professional clinician to find out what is right for you. Also, vitamin A supplements can be very dangerous to pregnant women and their developing babies and people with liver disease.

B Vitamins

The B vitamins are eight water-soluble vitamins that play important roles in cell metabolism. Historically, the B vitamins were once thought to be a single vitamin, referred to as vitamin B. Later research showed that there are eight chemically distinct vitamins that often coexist in the same foods. Supplements containing all eight B vitamins are generally referred to as a vitamin B complex. The B vitamins are:

- Vitamin B1 (Thiamine)
- Vitamin B2 (Riboflavin)
- Vitamin B3 (Niacin, includes nicotinic acid and nicotinamide)
- Vitamin B5 (Pantothenic acid)
- Vitamin B6 (Pyridoxine)
- Vitamin B7, also Vitamin H (Biotin)
- Vitamin B8 (myo-inositol) is no longer classified as a vitamin because it is synthesized by the human body
- Vitamin B9, also Vitamin M and Vitamin B-c (Folic acid)
- Vitamin B12 (Cobalamin)

The B vitamins often work together to deliver a number of health benefits to the body. B vitamins have been shown to:

- Support and increase the rate of metabolism;
- Maintain healthy skin and muscle tone;
- Enhance immune and nervous system function;

- Promote cell growth and division — including that of the red blood cells that help prevent anemia.

Vitamin B comes from a number of natural sources, including potatoes, bananas, lentils, chili peppers, tempeh, liver oil, liver, turkey, and tuna. Nutritional yeast (or brewer's yeast) and molasses are especially good sources of Vitamin B. I take B complex plus separate pills containing B1, B6 and B12.

B1 (Thiamine)

Vitamin B1 (Thiamine) is essential for normal growth and development and helps to maintain proper functioning of the heart and the nervous and digestive systems. Good food sources of thiamine include: brown rice, egg yolks, fish, legumes, liver, broccoli, and whole grains. The RDA for men is 1.2 mg (milligram) for men. Each day, I take 300 mg a day plus another 450 mg in a complex formula plus what I get from my B complex and multi-vitamin supplements. Therefore, I am taking well over 500 times the RDA. Again, this is what is right for me. To find out what is right for you, you should work with a professional clinician.

B2 (Riboflavin)

Vitamin B2 (Riboflavin) is required for a wide variety of cellular processes and plays a key role in energy metabolism. Milk, cheese, leafy green vegetables, liver, legumes such as mature soybeans, yeast and almonds are good sources of vitamin B2. I get 25 mg from my multivitamin. The RDA for adult males is 1.3 mg so I am consuming about 19 times the RDA.

B3 (Niacin)

Niacin, also known as nicotinic acid or vitamin B3, plays a number of critical roles in the body. Niacin or its derivatives are involved with detoxification, DNA repair, and the production of steroid hormones in the adrenal gland. Many different animal and plant foods can provide niacin including beef liver, brewer's yeast, broccoli, carrots, milk, wheat germ, and tomatoes. I get 125 mg through my multivitamin. The RDA is 16.

B5 (Pantothenic acid)

Pantothenic acid, also called vitamin B5, is involved in a wide array of key biological activities and is considered essential to all forms of life. Some people call it the "anti-stress vitamin" because it plays a role in the production of adrenal hormones. Good sources of vitamin B5 include: avocados, brewer's yeast, eggs, fresh vegetables, kidney, legumes, liver and saltwater fish. The "Adequate Intake" level for adults is 5 mg a day. I take 125 mg or 25 times the "Adequate Intake" level.

Vitamin B6 (Pyridoxine)

Pyridoxal phosphate is the active form of B6 and is a cofactor in many reactions of amino acid metabolism. In fact, it is thought to be involved in more bodily functions than almost any other single nutrient. Good food sources are brewer's yeast, carrots, eggs, fish, peas, spinach and wheat germ. The RDA is 1.3 or 1.7 mg for men depending on age. I take 200 mg a day and get an additional 50 mg in my multivitamin. This is nearly 150 times the RDA.

Vitamin B7 (Biotin)

Biotin is necessary for cell growth, the production of fatty acids, and the metabolism of fats and amino acids. Biotin is found in brewer's yeast, cooked egg yolks, saltwater fish, and whole grains. Thirty micrograms is considered an "Adequate Intake" for adults. I take 300 micrograms through my multivitamin or ten times the recommended allowance.

Vitamin B9 (Folic Acid)

Folic acid and folate are forms of the water-soluble Vitamin B9. Folic acid is needed for energy production and the formation of red blood cells. It is also necessary for healthy cell division. Leafy vegetables such as spinach and turnip greens, dried beans and peas, fortified cereal products, sunflower seeds and certain other fruits and vegetables, and liver are rich sources of folate. The RDA for adults is 400 microgram (mcg). I take 800 mcg twice each day plus 400 mcg in my once daily multivitamin. In total, I take five times the RDA.

Vitamin B12 (Cobalamin)

Vitamin B12 is important for the normal functioning of the brain and nervous system and for the formation of blood. It is involved in the metabolism of every cell of the body, especially affecting the DNA synthesis and regulation, but also fatty acid synthesis and energy production. Vitamin B12 is naturally found in foods of animal origin including meat (especially liver and shellfish) and milk products, and some sea vegetables (like kelp, kombu, and nori). The RDA for adults is 2.4 mcg. I take 5,000 mcg which is over two thousand times the RDA.

Vitamin C (Ascorbic Acid)

Unlike many animals, human beings cannot manufacture vitamin C and we must obtain it from diet or supplements. Vitamin C is found in citrus fruits, berries, and many green vegetables including: asparagus, avocados, broccoli, Brussels sprouts, and even onions.

Vitamin C has many key functions in the human body. It scavenges free radicals when it acts as an antioxidant, helps neutralize carcinogenic chemicals such as nitrosamine and nitrites, modulates cell growth and differentiation, and enhances the immune system by improving:

- lymphocyte function;
- the mobilization of phagocytes;
- natural killer cell activities;
- and immunoglobulin antibody levels.

Several of these mechanisms are directly related to the body's immune system and to cancer resistance. In fact, vitamin C is one of the most prevalent types of alternative and complimentary cancer therapy. Yet, this nutrient is still considered "controversial" by mainstream oncology.

The following information is excerpted from a Cancer News article published by Cancer Monthly. It summarizes some of the history about Vitamin C and cancer and discusses the pioneering work of Linus Pauling, Ph.D.

Almost all animals and plants synthesize their own vitamin C except humans and a small number of other animals, including, apes, guinea pigs, the red-vented bulbul, a fruit-eating bat and a species of trout.

Linus Pauling, Ph.D. (chemistry) had been interested in vitamin C for many years and had written previously how people required large amounts of vitamin C. Working with Dr. Cameron, Dr. Pauling pointed out that Vitamin C could: A) stimulate normal cells to produce increased amounts of a hyaluronidase inhibitor and; B) increase the number of collagen fibrils made. Based on these theories, Drs. Pauling and Cameron embarked on a number of studies to test the efficacy of vitamin C in cancer patients.

In 1976, Drs. Pauling and Cameron reported the survival times of 100 terminal cancer patients who were given supplemental ascorbate (10 grams/daily intravenously) and those of a control group of 1,000 patients of similar status treated by the same clinicians in the same hospital (Vale of Leven Hospital in Scotland) who had been managed identically except for the ascorbate. The 100 acorbate-treated patients lived, on the average, 300 days longer than their matched

37

controls with better quality of life (measured from the time all patients were considered "untreatable").

A second study was performed in 1978 with 100 new ascorbate-treated patients and 1,000 matched controls (about half of the controls were in the original set). This analysis broke out the improved survival times by cancer type. For each type of cancer there was an improvement in survival.

To test whether ascorbate was effective, Dr. Charles Moertel and his colleagues at the Mayo Clinic conducted two randomized placebo controlled studies of patients each with advanced cancer (published in 1979 and 1985). Patients randomized to the treatment group were given 10 grams of oral ascorbate, and neither study showed significant benefit. There were however, at least three significant differences between the Mayo Clinic's "definitive" studies and those of Drs. Pauling and Cameron.

The overwhelming majority - 87% (52 of 60 patients) of the patients in the first Mayo study had received chemotherapy before the study began. In contrast, only 4% of the patients in Pauling and Cameron study had received chemo. Pauling wrote, "It is known that cytotoxic chemotherapy damages the immune system and might prevent the vitamin C from being effective, inasmuch as it functions mainly by potentiating this system." (Note: in the 1985 Mayo clinic study, this difference was removed as none of the Mayo patients were administered prior chemotherapy.)

A commentary published by doctors from the National Institute of Health in 2000 pointed out that there was a second significant difference in study design that may have accounted for the different results in the Mayo Clinic studies. The authors explained that intravenous (IV) administration (used by Pauling and Cameron) was superior to oral administration (used by Moertel) in respect to bioavailability of the vitamin. The NIH authors said, "It is now clear that intravenous administration of ascorbate can yield very high plasma levels, while oral treatment does not." The NIH authors concluded that, "Moertel's results were not comparable to those of Cameron, as ascorbate was given orally and not intravenously. In retrospect, the route of administration may have been key."

This observation was repeated in another peer reviewed paper published in 2004 in the Annals of Internal Medicine which stated "Because efficacy of vitamin C treatment cannot be judged from clinical trials that use only oral dosing, the role of vitamin C in cancer treatment should be reevaluated."

And yet a third difference with the Mayo Clinic study was that vitamin C administration was discontinued immediately after a patient could no longer take oral medications or there was progression of the disease. Apparently, in the Pauling and Cameron studies vitamin C continued regardless of the patient's changing status. Vitamin C was provided during the life of the patient. However, in Moertel's studies, vitamin C was discontinued in a large number of patients whenever there was a sign of worsening. According to writer Ralph Moss, "Because of the odd departure from Cameron's protocol, patients in the treatment arm of the experiment (in Moertel's second study) received vitamin C for a median time of only 10 weeks. None of the Mayo patients died while receiving it. Their deaths occurred after the vitamin had been taken away from them."

Obviously if the Mayo Clinic studies were designed to test the outcomes of Drs. Pauling and Cameron studies then they should have replicated their methodology of administration (as long as it was scientifically reliable and clinically appropriate). Why didn't Moertel's group administer the vitamin intravenously throughout the life of the patient? We don't know. Any one of these discrepancies described above should have been sufficient for a complete reevaluation, but as is so often the case, the cancer establishment had successfully "proved" that a mere vitamin was of no value in cancer and the case was closed. Or was it?[18]

---

[18] Vitamin C and Cancer published by CancerWire, November 2006. Available here: http://www.cancermonthly.com/cancerwire/november2006

The article quoted above suggests that intravenous vitamin C may have more efficacy than oral vitamin C. I have only used the pill form, but many holistic doctors prefer to use the IV form on their cancer patients.

Whether Dr. Pauling was right or not will probably take years to decide. However, many cancer patients use vitamin C and many cancer clinics utilize it as a fundamental part of their protocol. I take eight grams of Vitamin C daily plus another gram from my multi-vitamins. The U.S. RDA for vitamin C for men over the age of 18 is 90 milligrams per day so I take 100 times more than the RDA. Nine grams may seem like a lot, but I know cancer patients who have taken five times what I consume (under a doctor's supervision, of course).

Generally with vitamin C there is something known as "bowel tolerance." Bowel tolerance basically means that your body will use as much vitamin C as it needs and after your consumption exceeds that amount you will have diarrhea. Therefore, under the care of a licensed clinician, one can use bowel tolerance as a guide to determine how much vitamin C your body may need. However, large doses of vitamin C can be dangerous to women who are pregnant. (According to some reports a developing infant may become dependant on the supplement and develop scurvy after being born.)

Vitamin D

Vitamin D is a group of fat-soluble pro-hormones, the two major forms of which are vitamin D2 (or ergocalciferol) and vitamin D3 (or cholecalciferol). Vitamin D plays a number of important roles in the human body including: maintaining organ systems; regulating calcium and phosphorus levels in the blood; promoting bone formation and mineralization and is essential in the development of an intact and strong skeleton; and promoting a strong immune system and anti-tumor activity. Good sources of vitamin D include: fish liver oils, saltwater fish, dairy products, and eggs. Vitamin D is also formed by the body in response to ultraviolet exposure.

According to the U.S. Government an "adequate intake" is 5 micrograms a day for men under 50 years of age, 10 micrograms from 51-70, and 15 micrograms for men over 70. I take 400 international units which substantially exceeds these levels. Note that without calcium, toxicity may result from taking too much supplemental vitamin D.

Vitamin E

Vitamin E is a fat-soluble vitamin that exists in eight different forms (all are called tocopherols or tocotrienols). Alpha-tocopherol (α-tocopherol) is the name of the most active form of vitamin E in humans.

Alpha-tocopherol acts as an antioxidant in humans. It prevents cell damage by inhibiting the oxidation of fats and the formation of free radicals. Vitamin E is found in many foods including: cold-pressed vegetable oils such as olive oil and soybean oil, brown rice, kelp, dark leafy vegetables, legumes, and whole grains. The RDA for adults for Vitamin E is 15 mg/day. I take over 400mg/day which is over 25 times the RDA.

Coenzyme Q10 (CoQ10)

Coenzyme Q10 (CoQ10) is a vitamin-like substance produced by the human body and is necessary for the basic functioning of cells. It is also powerful antioxidant. CoQ10 levels are reported to decrease with age and to be low in patients with some chronic diseases such as heart conditions, muscular dystrophies, cancer, diabetes, and HIV/AIDS. CoQ10 can be found in many foods including mackerel, salmon, sardines and spinach. I take 120 mg twice a day.

Minerals

All life on the planet depends on minerals for proper functioning and structure. Minerals are needed for the composition of body fluids, formation of blood and bone, and maintenance of nerve function. Nutritionally, minerals belong to two groups: macrominerals and trace minerals.

Macrominerals include calcium, magnesium, sodium, potassium, and phosphorus. Trace minerals, which are needed in smaller amounts, include boron, chromium, copper, germanium, iodine, iron, selenium, zinc, and others.

Macrominerals

Calcium

Calcium is one of the most abundant elements on Earth, and it is the most abundant mineral in the human body. It performs many important roles including controlling muscle contractions, initiating DNA synthesis, and building bones. Calcium can be found in dairy foods, various seafood, dark leafy vegetables, and many other foods. I take 250 mg a day through my multivitamin. An "adequate intake" is considered 1,000 mg to 1,300 mg. depending on age, so I only get about 25% through my supplements. I am confident, however, that I get enough because calcium is present in many of the foods I eat.

Magnesium

Magnesium is the fourth most abundant mineral in the body and is essential to good health. Magnesium is needed for many critical functions in the body including: maintaining normal muscle and nerve function, keeping the heart rhythm steady, supporting a healthy immune system, and helping to maintain bone strength, regulating blood sugar levels, and promoting normal blood pressure. Green vegetables such as spinach are good sources of magnesium. The RDA for adult males depends on age and ranges from 400 to 420 milligrams a day. I take 125 milligrams in my supplements and get the rest through my diet.

Potassium

Potassium is an essential dietary mineral and electrolyte that is needed for nerve function, muscle contraction and maintenance of normal blood pressure. Potassium is also important for chemical reactions within the body and regulates the transfer of nutrients through cell membranes. Good sources of potassium include dairy foods, fish, fruit, legumes, and whole grains. I take 800 grams per day. The U.S. Government's "adequate intake" for Potassium in adults is 4.7 grams per day so I take over 170 times this amount.

Trace Minerals

Chromium

Chromium is a mineral that humans require in trace amounts. It is found primarily in two forms: 1) trivalent (chromium 3+), which is biologically active and found in food, and 2) hexavalent (chromium 6+), a toxic form that results from industrial pollution. The non-toxic biologically active form is needed in the metabolism of glucose. (Therefore, if you have diabetes chromium supplementation can be dangerous.) Meat and whole-grain products, as well as some fruits and vegetables are considered good sources of this trace mineral. The "adequate intake" amount is 35 micrograms for adult males. I take 120 micrograms.

Copper

Copper is an essential trace nutrient. In animals and people it is found primarily in the bloodstream, as a co-factor in various enzymes, and in copper-based pigments. Among its many functions, copper assists in the formation of bone, hemoglobin, and red blood cells. It is believed that zinc and copper compete for absorption in the digestive tract so that a diet that is excessive in one of these minerals may result in a deficiency in the other.

Trace amounts of copper can be found in many foods including: avocados, barley, beans, beets, broccoli, garlic and green leafy vegetables. The RDA for copper in adults is approximately 900 micrograms a day. I get 2 milligrams from my multivitamin.

Iodine

Iodine is an essential trace element and is a critical constituent of the thyroid hormones, thyroxine (T4) and triiodothyronine (T3). These hormones play a critical role in human biology and act on gene transcription and basal metabolic rate. Iodine also helps to metabolize excess fat and is needed for mental development. The RDA for adults is 150 micrograms per day. I get this exact amount through my multivitamin. Note that excessive iodine can actually inhibit the secretion of thyroid hormone. Foods that contain iodine include: iodized salts, seafood, saltwater fish, and kelp.

Iron

Iron is one of the most abundant metals on Earth and is vital to human physiology. In humans, iron is an essential component of proteins involved in oxygen transport and for the regulation of cell growth. Almost two-thirds of iron in the body is found in hemoglobin, the protein in red blood cells that carries oxygen to tissues. Iron can be found in red meats, fish, and poultry, lentils and beans. I take 800 micrograms a day through my multivitamin. The RDA is 8 mg for a male over 18 years of age so I am getting 10% of the RDA. However, like Calcium, my nutritionist believes I am getting sufficient iron through my normal diet. Iron deficiency symptoms may include anemia, brittle hair, difficulty swallowing, dizziness, and fatigue.

Manganese

Manganese is an essential trace nutrient in all forms of life and is involved in many enzyme reactions including protein and fat metabolism. It is also needed for a healthy immune system. Good sources of manganese include: avocados, nuts and seeds, seaweed, and whole grains. The "adequate intake" for an adult male is 2.3 milligrams per day. I take 4 milligrams per day.

Selenium

Selenium is a trace mineral that is essential to good health. It is incorporated into proteins to make selenoproteins, which are important antioxidant enzymes that prevent cellular damage from free radicals. It is thought that selenium and vitamin E act together to aid in the production of antibodies. Selenium can be found in Brazil nuts, brewer's yeast, broccoli, brown rice, kelp, and many other foods. Generally, the content of selenium in food depends on the selenium content of the soil where the food is grown. Selenium also can be found in some meats and seafood. An "adequate intake" is 55 micrograms for adults. I take 70 micrograms through my multivitamin.

Zinc

Zinc is an essential element, necessary for sustaining all life. It is important in prostate gland functioning and the growth of the reproductive organs. Zinc is also an activator of certain enzymes and also promotes a healthy immune system. Zinc is found in brewer's yeast, fish, kelp, legumes, liver, and many other foods. The RDA for zinc is adult males is 11 milligrams a day. I take 15 milligrams daily.

Amino Acids

Amino acids are the building blocks of proteins. Every living organism from human beings to the tiniest bacteria are composed of proteins. After water, proteins make up the greatest part of our body weight. Proteins are what make our muscles, ligaments, organs, glands, nails, hair, and various fluids. In addition, all the enzymes that act as catalysts to maintain life are proteins.

There are 20 amino acids. Humans can produce 10 of them. The others must be supplied in the food. The 10 amino acids that we can produce ("nonessential") are alanine, asparagine, aspartic acid, cysteine, glutamic acid, glutamine, glycine, proline, serine and tyrosine. Tyrosine is produced from phenylalanine, so if the diet is deficient in phenylalanine, tyrosine will be required as well.

The essential amino acids (the ones we can't produce) are arginine, histidine, isoleucine, leucine, lysine, methionine, phenylalanine, threonine, tryptophan, and valine. Unlike fat and starch, the human body does not store excess amino acids for later use—the amino acids must be in the food every day. Failure to obtain enough of even one of the ten essential amino acids, those that we cannot make, can result in degradation of the body's proteins. I get all of the essential amino acids in my multivitamin and most of the nonessential ones as well.

Herbs

I also consume a number of herbs and herbal products. One in particular is called Essiac. Essiac is not an herb itself, but a tea comprised of a blend of herbs.

Essiac Tea has been used by cancer patients since the 1930's. The tea was first formulated by a Canadian nurse, Rene Caisse, who named it after her last name spelled backwards. The original formula is believed to have its roots in native Canadian Ojibwa medicine. The basic components of the tea include greater burdock root (Arctium lappa), slippery elm inner bark (Ulmus rubra), sheep sorrel (Rumex acetosella), and Indian or Turkish rhubarb root (Rheum officinale). Although, there is some debate over which formula is more effective, and which one is "authentic," many cancer patients have used one form or another for over half a century. I drink Essiac Tea (two ounces twice a day.) One ounce first thing in the morning and one ounce just prior to going to bed.

Burdock

Burdock is one of the ingredients of Essiac Tea. Burdock is a thistle that grows wild throughout most of North America, Europe and Asia. Folk herbalists consider dried burdock to be a diuretic, diaphoretic, and a blood purifying agent. The seeds of greater burdock are used in traditional Chinese medicine, under the name niupangzi. Modern research has revealed that burdock has antioxidant properties. (Note: Burdock can interfere with iron absorption and should not be used by: pregnant or breast feeding women, diabetics, or people with cardiovascular conditions.)

Slippery Elm

Slippery Elm is a tree native to eastern North America. It was traditionally used by Native Americans as a poultice for boils, ulcers and for wounds in general. Internally, it was commonly used for colds or fevers and to soothe an irritated digestive system – one of its main uses today. The plant contains mucilage, a long chain of sugars (polysaccharides) that make a slippery substance when combined with water. This mucilage is believed to soothe the digestive system.

Sheep Sorrel

Sheep Sorrel is a common perennial weed that is native to Eurasia but has been introduced to most of the rest of the northern hemisphere. At least ten Native American tribes in Canada and the United States have used this plant, also known as sour grass or sour weed, as a food or medicine. Sheep sorrel is a popular ingredient of many folk remedies and the tea was used traditionally as a diuretic and to treat fevers, inflammation and scurvy. Based on reports by Rene Caisse and her clinician colleagues who performed studies with mice bearing abnormal

47

growths, sheep sorrel is considered the most active herb in Essiac for stimulating cellular regeneration, detoxification and cleansing.

Turkish Rhubarb Root

Turkish Rhubarb, a type of perennial plant, has been used traditionally to improve both digestion and loss of appetite. The bitter tea is rich in tannins that increase the flow of saliva and gastric secretions and can reportedly be used as an astringent or stomachic at a low dosage to stop diarrhea. There are some peer reviewed medical articles that suggest Rheum palmatum is anti-cancer in a cell line and anti-viral (Hepatitis B).

Fenu-Thyme

I also take Fenu-Thyme which is a supplement that contains two herbs – Fenugreek and Thyme.

Fenugreek is an ancient medicinal herb that has been used for a variety of health conditions, including digestive problems, constipation, and reducing mucus. It is also thought to reduce fever.

Thyme is thought to also reduce fever, and lessen headaches and mucus. In addition, the essential oil of common thyme is comprised of 20-55% thyol which is a powerful antiseptic.

Food Supplements

I also consume a number of natural food supplements. These often contain concentrates from specific fruits or vegetables. There is a great deal of variety with these products. Many health food stores carry dozens of different types and brands. Keep in mind that the potency of these products varies. Since they are comprised of essentially perishable foods their potency is affected by shelf life, temperature and other variables.

Here are some that I take:

Artichoke – a good source of potassium and antioxidants.

Grapefruit Pectin – a good source of fiber

Grape seed with resveratrol – This grape seed product contains proanthocyanidins (a powerful antioxidant) and other flavonoids. Flavonoids have been shown to be anti-allergic, anti-inflammatory, anti-microbial and may have anti-cancer activity. In addition, grapeseed oil contains a large amount of linoleic acid.

Beta glucan – Beta glucans are polysaccharides occurring in the bran of cereal grains, the cell wall of baker's yeast, certain types of fungi, and many kinds of mushrooms. They are thought to have anti-cancer properties.

Maitake Mushroom - Maitake is an edible mushroom from the species Grifola frondosa. Research has shown that a maitake extract (maitake D-fraction) has immune system effects in animal and laboratory studies. I take 1/2 eye dropper twice a day when I feel that my mesothelioma may be recurring.

Acidophilus – Acidophilus is a general name for a group of probiotics, often added to milk or sold as a capsule, which may contain: Lactobacillus acidophilus, Lactobacillus casei, Lactobacillus bulgaricus, Bifidobacterium species, and Streptococcus thermophilus. These "friendly" bacteria inhabit the intestines and protect against the entrance and proliferation of "bad" organisms that can cause disease. The primary dietary sources of L. acidophilus include milk enriched with acidophilus, yogurt containing live L. acidophilus cultures, miso, and tempeh. I take one gram, two times a day.

Antioxidants

I also take a number of supplements that are known for their antioxidant properties. These include:

Alpha Lipoic Acid – Alpha lipoic acid is a strong antioxidant.

Lycopene - Lycopene is a bright red carotenoid pigment found in tomatoes and other red fruits. Lycopene is the most common carotenoid in the human body and is a potent antioxidant. In addition, it is considered a promising agent for prostate cancer prevention. I take 20 mg a day.

L-glutathione – Glutathione is a peptide molecule synthesized in the body from the three amino acids and is one of the body's most important and powerful antioxidants. I take 100 milligrams three times a day.

ঙ 4 ঙ

Nutrition & Mesothelioma:
The Vitamin A Example

ANY DOCTOR WHO TELLS YOU THAT DIET, VITAMINS, AND OTHER HOLISTIC CONSIDERATIONS PLAY NO ROLE IN THE PREVENTION OR MANAGEMENT OF CANCER, OR MESOTHELIOMA IN PARTICULAR, IS EITHER IGNORANT OR WORSE. Yes, a great deal more research is needed to "prove" the therapeutic value of these natural modalities. But while the years go by and we wait for things to get "proven" people are dying.

How much research is necessary before a vitamin or any natural approach is considered beneficial to managing mesothelioma or any other cancer? How much is enough? In this example, I report some of what science already knows about mesothelioma and vitamin A. This information is taken directly from the scientific/medical literature, the journals written and read by our doctors and medical experts. As you will read there is already some scientific evidence that suggests that the various forms of vitamin A may be beneficial to mesothelioma patients or people who want to avoid getting the disease.

Let's be clear – I am not suggesting that vitamin A is either a cure or prevention for mesothelioma. I am just relaying what some scientists have reported.

Remember that the same caveat always applies – if you are interested in using these types of approaches don't do it on your own. Work with an experienced and licensed professional

51

clinician. Vitamin A, in the wrong amounts, can actually be dangerous.

Vitamin A and Mesothelioma

Study #1) Low levels of retinol have been associated with an increased risk of developing mesothelioma.

In this study, Australian researchers looked at former workers and residents exposed to crocidolite (blue asbestos) in Western Australia. Their findings suggested that "people with chronically low plasma levels of retinol (the fat-soluble animal form of vitamin A found in liver and eggs) have increased risk of developing mesothelioma and lung cancer."[19] This is a fascinating conclusion. It implies that a person's intake of retinol or perhaps other forms of vitamin A may affect their vulnerability to mesothelioma.

Study #2) Cruciferous vegetables and carotene may make mesothelioma less likely.

In a 1988 study in Louisiana performed by the National Cancer Institute, the dietary patterns of mesothelioma patients were compared to those of healthy individuals.[20] According to

---

[19] "Increased rates of death from asbestos-related diseases have been reported in former workers and residents exposed to crocidolite (blue asbestos) at Wittenoom (Western Australia). The relationships between plasma concentrations of retinol, carotene and vitamin E and incidence of mesothelioma and lung cancer in a cohort of people from this town were examined…These findings suggest that people with chronically low plasma levels of retinol have increased risk of developing mesothelioma and lung cancer." Source: Alfonso HS, et al., Plasma vitamin concentrations and incidence of mesothelioma and lung cancer in individuals exposed to crocidolite at Wittenoom, Western Australia. Eur J Cancer Prev. 2006 Aug;15(4):290-4.

[20] Schiffman MH, et al., Case-control study of diet and mesothelioma in Louisiana. Cancer Res. 1988 May 15;48 (10):2911-5

the article, mesothelioma patients ate less homegrown, cruciferous vegetables and all vegetables combined *before they were diagnosed* compared to healthy patients. Cruciferous vegetables, also called Brassica Vegetables, include Arugula, Broccoli, Cauliflower, Brussels Sprouts, Cabbage, Watercress, Bok Choy, Turnip Greens, Kale, and Mustard Greens. The researchers also pointed out that carotene intake was significantly lower for the mesothelioma patients. Carotene is a precursor to vitamin A. This suggests, once again, that diet and vitamin A in particular may affect the onset of mesothelioma.

Study #3) Vitamin A or beta-carotene may decrease the risk of mesothelioma.

In this 1996 study from the Division of Epidemiology of the American Health Foundation, the investigators examined the association between dietary intake and mesothelioma by studying 94 men and women with malignant mesothelioma and 64 people without cancer. They concluded that their results provided "some justification for the hypothesis that provitamin A or beta-carotene may decrease the risk of mesothelioma."[21] Provitamin A is any of the carotenoids that are precursors of vitamin A and can be found in fish-liver oils, egg yolk, milk products, green-leaf or yellow vegetables, and fruits.

Study #4) Retinoic Acid may make mesothelioma less likely to metastasize.

---

[21] "A high consumption of fruit and vegetables reduces the risk of several types of cancer. There is little information on the association between dietary intake and mesothelioma. A hospital-based case-control study of 94 men and women with malignant mesothelioma and 64 control patients without cancer was conducted to determine the odds associated with consumption of carotenoid-containing fruits and vegetables...These results provide some justification for the hypothesis that provitamin A or beta-carotene may decrease the risk of mesothelioma." Source: Muscat JE, Huncharek M. Dietary intake and the risk of malignant mesothelioma. Br J Cancer. 1996 May;73(9):1122-5.

In a study from 2002, researchers looked at mesothelioma cells *in vitro* (in test tubes or Petri dishes outside the body) and found that retinoic acid (the oxidized form of Vitamin A) "may lead to a decrease of mesothelioma cell local invasion." They interpreted this to mean that retinoic acid may modify how mesothelioma grows and spreads in the body.[22] This study suggests that vitamin A levels may actually affect the aggressiveness of mesothelioma once someone is diagnosed with the disease.

How many mesothelioma patients or people exposed to asbestos are given this information by their doctors? None that I have ever spoken to. To be fair, this is very preliminary research. These studies, however, suggest that vitamin A may be of benefit to people with mesothelioma or those who want to avoid getting the disease in the first place. In a disease like this where treatment options are limited and people are searching for answers, this information, although preliminary, can be of value.

Will we ever know if mesothelioma patients should be routinely prescribed vitamin A and in what amounts? How much current research is being conducted into this question? Currently, there are no clinical trials or studies according to the National Cancer Institute. Therefore, if you want to take vitamin A or a form of vitamin A in one of various supplements you should be under the care of a licensed clinician.

---

[22]Scarpa S, et al., Retinoic acid inhibits fibronectin and laminin synthesis and cell migration of human pleural mesothelioma in vitro. Oncol Rep. 2002 Jan-Feb;9(1):205-9.

ഌ 5 ര

Cancer, Nutrition and the Scientific Evidence

VITAMIN A IS NOT THE ONLY EXAMPLE OF A NUTRIENT THAT MAY BE OF BENEFIT TO PATIENTS WITH CANCER OR MESOTHELIOMA IN PARTICULAR. There are actually thousands of scientific studies that have concluded that there may be benefits from various dietary, vitamin and herbal approaches to cancer. However, many of these results come from cell culture studies and animal models, not human clinical studies.

In fact, you may get slightly annoyed like I was when you read that some of these studies were performed five, ten, or more than 15 years ago. You may wonder why so little progress has been made to test these compounds in patients when positive laboratory results have been known for decades. The answer is economic, not scientific.

As previously discussed, these natural agents are difficult to patent (a company may be able to patent the manufacturing process, but not the compound itself.) This is because these are naturally occurring agents and they were not invented by a drug company. Since they were not invented by the pharmaceutical industry and are therefore difficult to patent (you can't patent something you didn't invent), drug companies will not spend the reported 500 million dollars or more needed to complete human clinical testing. This is understandable. Why would any profit making company invest millions of dollars of their own money to prove that something works in cancer when they cannot make any money from it. For example, if a drug company paid for clinical testing that demonstrated that vitamin A or certain herbs or mushrooms were more effective than chemotherapy in treating mesothelioma where would that leave them? Anyone could buy the vitamins for a couple of dollars and grow the mushrooms or herbs on their windowsill or in their backyard. Chemotherapy sales would plummet. From an economic standpoint this would be a very bad decision indeed. And, of course, companies are driven by economics.

To give you an idea of how much science already knows about natural compounds and cancer, I have included some examples from the scientific literature. This is just the tip of the iceberg. There are thousands of studies like these. Obviously what may be potentially effective in melanoma or liver cancer or colon cancer may not be effective is mesothelioma. Nevertheless, it is instructive to see positive results that have been obtained when cancer cells (in test tubes, animals, or sometimes in people) are exposed to various nutrients.

Remember that the same caveat always applies – if you are interested in using these types of approaches don't do it on your own. Work with an experienced and licensed professional clinician.

Vitamin B6 kills rate liver cancer cells and human kidney cancer cells in cultures

In 1982 researchers found that vitamin B6 (pyridoxine) "can retard and eventually kill Fu5-5 rat liver cancer cells in culture." They also found a similar effect in a human cancer kidney cell line. The researchers concluded that "These findings suggest the potential use of vitamin B6 as an antineoplastic [anti-cancer] agent."[23]

---

[23] DiSorbo DM and Litwack G., Vitamin B6 kills hepatoma cells in culture. Nutr Cancer. 1982;3(4):216-22.

Vitamin E, beta-carotene and selenium decrease mortality rate from stomach cancer

In 2000, researchers found that vitamin E, beta-carotene and selenium "significantly decreased mortality rate from stomach cancer...and showed signs of other beneficial effects."[24]

Folate, vitamins B6, B12, E, and C, and selenium are protective against colorectal cancer

In 2006 researchers in Australia examined dietary factors associated with colorectal cancer risk.[25] They found that folate (a form of vitamin B9) protected against rectal cancer and vitamin B6 and B12 consumption was protective for both colon and rectal cancer. They also found that dietary selenium was significantly protective at both cancer sites. In addition, they found that vitamins E and C were "significantly protective for both colon and rectal cancer at all levels of consumption, and for both vitamins there was a dose-response effect of increasing protection, particularly so for colon cancer. In other words, the more vitamin E and C these people took, the less likely they were to be diagnosed with colon or rectal cancer.

Healthy nutrient mixture reduces mesothelioma cells ability to invade

---

[24] Yang CS., Vitamin nutrition and gastroesophageal cancer. J Nutr. 2000 Feb;130(2S Suppl):338S-339S.

[25] Kune G, Watson L., Colorectal cancer protective effects and the dietary micronutrients folate, methionine, vitamins B6, B12, C, E, selenium, and lycopene. : Nutr Cancer. 2006;56(1):11-21

In 2006, researchers created a mixture of lysine, proline, ascorbic acid, and green tea extract.[26] Lysine is an essential amino acid (humans cannot synthesize it). Proline is an amino acid, but not an essential amino acid, which means that humans can synthesize it. Ascorbic acid is a sugar acid with antioxidant properties. One form of ascorbic acid is commonly known as vitamin C. And green tea contains many substances thought to be beneficial including a number of antioxidants. The researchers exposed a mesothelioma cell line to this mixture and found that it reduced the cancer cells ability to invade. This again hints that certain natural compounds may be able to reduce the metastatic ability of mesothelioma in people.

The Reishi mushroom (Ganoderma lucidum) enables premalignant bladder cells to die in culture

Researchers tested the reishi mushroom *Ganoderma lucidum* *in vitro* (in a model of human premalignant urothelial cells) and found that it induced apoptosis (cell suicide) in these cells. The authors concluded that their "study strongly suggests that *G. lucidum* is a potential source of chemopreventive agents for bladder cancer based on its effectiveness in controlling the premalignant urothelial cell growth and carcinogen-induced transformation."[27]

Mango combats testosterone-induced changes in mouse prostate

Mango pulp extract and Lupeol (an ingredient of mango and other fruits) were tested in mouse prostate cancer. These

---

[26] Roomi MW, et al., Inhibition of malignant mesothelioma cell matrix metalloproteinase production and invasion by a novel nutrient mixture. Exp Lung Res. 2006 Mar-Apr;32(3-4):69-79.

[27] John W., et al., Telomerase-Associated Apoptotic Events by Mushroom Ganoderma lucidum on Premalignant Human Urothelial Cells, Nutrition and Cancer, Volume 60, Issue 1 January 2008, pages 109 – 119.

animals were first injected with testosterone. The researchers concluded that the Mango pulp extract and Lupeol combination "is effective in combating testosterone-induced changes in mouse prostate..."[28]

Lycopene and soy isoflavones stabilized PSA levels in men with prostate cancer

In 2007 researchers administered a tomato extract capsule (containing 15 milligrams of lycopene) alone or in combination with a capsule containing 40 milligrams of a soy isoflavone (a type of flavonoid) to men with prostate cancer and rising PSA levels. The compounds were administered twice daily orally for a maximum of 6 months. The researchers found that 95% of the patients in the lycopene group and 67% patients in the lycopene plus soy isoflavone group had stable PSA levels. The scientists concluded, "The data suggest that lycopene and soy isoflavones...may delay progression of both hormone-refractory and hormone-sensitive prostate cancer."[29]

Vitamins B2 and B6 levels "significantly lower" in lung cancer patients

In 2007 researchers looked at vitamin B levels in red blood cells of patients with non-small cell lung cancer (NSCLC). They found that, "Vitamins B2 and B6 levels in red blood cells (RBC) from NSCLC patients were significantly lower [than healthy

---

[28] Sahdeo Prasad, et al., Induction of Apoptosis by Lupeol and Mango Extract in Mouse Prostate and LNCaP Cells, Nutrition and Cancer, Volume 60, Issue 1 January 2008, pages 120 – 130.

[29] Ulka Vaishampayan, et al., Lycopene and Soy Isoflavones in the Treatment of Prostate Cancer Nutrition and Cancer, Volume 59, Issue 1 September 2007 , pages 1 – 7.

people]." They concluded that, "the importance of vitamins B2 and B6 for NSCLC patients could not be ignored."[30]

Vitamin E suppresses mammary tumor growth in rats

In this study, rats were fed a carcinogen (N-methyl-N-nitrosourea) and then fed mixed tocopherols. (Vitamin E is the collective name for a set of eight related tocopherols and tocotrienols.) The researchers found that "dietary administration of mixed tocopherols significantly suppressed mammary tumor growth."[31]

Docosahexaenoic acid (DHA) inhibits colon carcinoma (in a mouse model)

Docosahexaenoic acid (DHA) is an omega-3 essential fatty acid. When it was fed to mice with human colon carcinoma cells it inhibited tumor growth by 93%. DHA is most often found in fish oil.[32]

Black tea helps the immune system recognize Ehrlich's ascites carcinoma in mice

Cancer has been found to impair a host's immune function. Researchers found that black tea helped to stop this impairment

---

[30] Shih-Ming Tsao, et al., Oxidant Stress and B Vitamins Status in Patients With Non-Small Cell Lung Cancer, Nutrition and Cancer, Volume 59, Issue 1 September 2007, pages 8 – 13.

[31] Nanjoo Suh, et al., Mixed Tocopherols Inhibit N-methyl-N-Nitrosourea-Induced Mammary Tumor Growth in Rats Nutrition and Cancer, Volume 59, Issue 1 September 2007, pages 76 – 81.

[32] Taeko Kato, et al. Docosahexaenoic Acid (DHA), a Primary Tumor Suppressive Omega-3 Fatty Acid, Inhibits Growth of Colorectal Cancer Independent of p53 Mutational Status. Nutrition and Cancer, Volume 58, Issue 2 July 2007, pages 178 – 187.

when they tested the tea in Ehrlich's ascites carcinoma (EAC)-bearing mice.[33]

Lack of Vitamin D associated with cancer

In 2006 researchers examined Vitamin D levels in 70 cancer patients. They found that 72% were deficient in this vitamin. The researchers concluded that deficiency of vitamin D "could play a role in cancer development and host response to tumor and therapy."[34]

Flaxseed meal reduces colon cancer in rats

Flaxseed meal or corn meal was fed to rats that were injected with a carcinogen. The rats who received flaxseed meal had over 50% less tumors and the tumors they did have were much smaller, about 10% the size of the tumors in the corn meal fed rats. The researchers concluded that in their study, dietary flaxseed meal was effective in preventing colon tumor development when compared with dietary corn meal.[35]

---

[33] Debaprasad Mandal, et al. Black Tea-Induced Decrease in IL-10 and TGF-b.beta of Tumor Cells Promotes Th1/Tc1 Response in Tumor Bearer. Nutrition and Cancer, Volume 58, Issue 2 July 2007, pages 213 – 221.

[34] Ashley Serene Plant and Glenn Tisman, Frequency of Combined Deficiencies of Vitamin D and Holotranscobalamin in Cancer Patients. Nutrition and Cancer, Volume 56, Issue 2 January 2006, pages 143 – 148.

[35] Ajay Bommareddy, et al. Chemopreventive Effects of Dietary Flaxseed on Colon Tumor Development. Nutrition and Cancer, Volume 54, Issue 2 January 2006, pages 216 – 222.

ಜಿ 6 ೲ

CASE STUDIES

I DO NOT ADVOCATE THAT PATIENTS WITH MESOTHELIOMA OR ANY OTHER CANCER REJECT CONVENTIONAL THERAPIES LIKE CHEMOTHERAPY, RADIATION OR SURGERY. I just believe that when these conventional therapies have little to offer that patients should examine all their options.

How often do cancer patients like me decide to reject conventional cancer therapies such as radiation and chemotherapy and use nutritional holistic therapies instead? Probably quite a few, especially when the conventional therapies offer little hope. How often do thee patients actually benefit? I do not know. Obviously it depends on many variables – the type of cancer, the kind of therapies, whether or not the patient was overseen by professional clinicians, etc. I have no doubt that many patients who use alternative therapies get some benefit in their quality of life. There may be lessening of pain or an increase in appetite or energy. But, how many patients actually survive their cancer longer because of alternative therapies and approaches? This is an important question that has never been answered in a comprehensive fashion. No study has been performed. Instead we have anecdotes and case studies. Here are five examples of cancer patients who enjoyed a surprising benefit from alternative approaches. Their stories have been written up as case histories in the medical literature by doctors and researchers.

Fish and Algae Oils Make Sarcoma Nodules Decrease in 78 Year Old Man

This first case is about a 78 year old man with malignant fibrous histiocytoma with multiple lesions in both lungs.[36] Malignant fibrous histiocytoma (MFH) is the most common soft tissue sarcoma of late adult life. After this patient was diagnosed, "he declined conventional chemotherapy and elected nutritional intervention by increasing intake of omega-3 fatty acids and lowering intake of omega-6 fatty acids." The authors of this case study estimated that this patient consumed 15 grams of the long-chain omega-3 fatty acids eicosapentaenoic (EPA) and docosahexaenoic acid (DHA) per day. According to the doctors, CAT scans and X-rays "revealed remarkably a slow and steady decrease in the size and number of bilateral nodules. He has no apparent side effects from consuming large quantities of fish and algae oils rich in DHA and EPA and he remains asymptomatic."

So here is a 78 year old man who ate "large quantities of fish and algae oils" and made his sarcoma nodules decrease slowly and steadily.

Reishi Mushroom May Have Made Lymphoma Cells Disappear in 47 Year Old Patient

In this case report, a 47-year-old man was diagnosed with a high-grade lymphoma (B-cell lymphoma) by biopsy.[37] Eleven days later "no evidence was found of large B-cell lymphoma despite thorough sampling." Instead the doctors found immense

---

[36] Ronald S. Pardini, et al., Nutritional Intervention With Omega-3 Fatty Acids in a Case of Malignant Fibrous Histiocytoma of the Lungs. Nutrition and Cancer, Volume 52, Issue 2 July 2005, pages 121 – 129.

[37] Cheuk W, et al., Regression of gastric large B-Cell lymphoma accompanied by a florid lymphoma-like T-cell reaction: immunomodulatory effect of Ganoderma lucidum (Lingzhi)? Int J Surg Pathol. 2007 Apr;15(2):180-6.

populations of T cells. T cells are a type of white blood cell that play a key role in our immune system. The doctors questioned the patient as to what we had been doing in the past few days. The patient explained that he had been consuming "megadoses of *Ganoderma lucidum.*" *Ganoderma lucidum* is a mushroom that also goes by the name of reishi. According to the authors of the case study, "*Ganoderma lucidum* might have triggered the successful immune reaction."

Chinese Herbs May Have Contributed to Regression of Lung Cancer in 51 Year Old Women

A 51-year-old woman was diagnosed with squamous cell carcinoma (SCC) of the lung.[38] It was staged T2N2M0. Eight years later she had a "complete regression of her lung carcinoma." According to the researchers that wrote the case study the woman "had been treated with Chinese herbal medicine alone for 4 years. The herbal prescription consisted of nine Chinese medicinal herbs. These herbs have been reported to possess anti-tumor and immune enhancing effects. Therefore, it is suggested that the herbal treatment for this patient might have contributed to the complete regression of her lung carcinoma. Further research on the actions of these herbs is warranted."

Terminal Pancreatic Cancer Patient Recovers with Lipoic Acid, Healthy Lifestyle Program and a Drug

In this case study the authors describe the long-term survival of a patient with pancreatic cancer.[39] The treatment regimen included:

---

[38] Liang HL, et al., Regression of squamous cell carcinoma of the lung by Chinese herbal medicine: a case with an 8-year follow-up. Lung Cancer. 2004 Mar;43(3):355-60.

[39] Berkson BM, et al., The long-term survival of a patient with pancreatic cancer with metastases to the liver after treatment with the intravenous alpha-lipoic acid/low-dose naltrexone protocol. Integr Cancer Ther. 2006 Mar;5(1):83-9.

1) Intravenous alpha-lipoic acid. (Lipoic acid is an organic compound which is an essential cofactor for many enzyme complexes.)
2) Low-dose naltrexone (ALA-N) protocol. (Naltrexone is a drug used primarily in the management of alcohol dependence.)
3) And a healthy lifestyle program.

The authors of the study wrote: "The patient was told by a reputable university oncology center in October 2002 that there was little hope for his survival. Today, January 2006, however, he is back at work, free from symptoms, and without appreciable progression of his malignancy. The integrative protocol described in this article may have the possibility of extending the life of a patient who would be customarily considered to be terminal...Several other patients are on this treatment protocol and appear to be doing well at this time."

Gerson Therapy Benefits 34 Year Old Women with Brain Cancer

The Gerson therapy consists of flooding the body with nutrients from about 20 pounds of organically grown fresh fruits and vegetables on a daily basis.

In 1996 a 34-year old woman was diagnosed with a recurrent anaplastic astrocytoma (an aggressive brain cancer).[40] The cancer had returned after radiation therapy. The woman started on the Gerson therapy. A review in June 1997 showed that there was no evidence of any active tumor in the surrounding area of the brain. A review in November 1998 also showed no increase in size. In 1999, the Gerson regimen was scaled down (maintenance phase of the Gerson regimen), and the homeopathic remedy pulsatilla was added. A review in

---

[40] Molassiotis A and Peat P. Surviving against all odds: analysis of 6 case studies of patients with cancer who followed the Gerson therapy. Integr Cancer Ther. 2007 Mar;6(1):80-8.

November 2000 showed no increase in size from the previous year. She has since had annual reviews with still no increase in tumor size, although symptoms of headaches and seizures continued throughout. According to the case study, "The patient remains well and stable at present."

These anecdotes or case stories merely whet our appetite that some alternative approaches in some patients may actually be highly effective. But, we know so little. We don't know what happened to their immune systems because they were not tested or monitored. We don't know why these approaches did what they did. It's not because we don't have the technology to answer these questions. It's really because mainstream cancer care is not interested in knowing. No one is testing me to see how or why I have survived so long.

ഒ 7 ര

MIND BODY MEDICINE

IF WHAT WE EAT CAN NOURISH OUR BODY, WHAT WE THINK CAN NOURISH OUR MIND. Mind-body medicine focuses on the powerful ways in which emotional, mental, spiritual, and behavioral factors can directly affect our health.

The concept that the mind is important in healing disease is not a "new age" idea. In fact, it may be considered traditional medicine because it has been around for more than 2,000 years in Greek, Chinese and Ayurvedic medicine. The Greek physician Hippocrates, considered the "father of medicine," recognized the moral and spiritual aspects of healing, and believed that treatment could occur only with consideration of attitude, environmental influences, and natural remedies. While this integrated approach was maintained in traditional healing systems in the East, developments in the Western world by the 16th and 17th centuries led to a separation of human spiritual and emotional dimensions from the physical body.

During the Enlightenment era, a Reductionist perspective became popular in which the human body was regarded as a machine like a clock. Because the emphasis was on the mechanical, anything that could not be seen and quantified was considered not to exist. These early scientists saw no physical proof of the connection between the spiritual and emotional dimensions and the physical body. The separation of mind from matter and body was complete...for a time.

The Placebo Effect

During World War II, the importance of belief reentered the concept of health care. On the beaches of Anzio in Italy, morphine for the wounded soldiers was in short supply, and Henry Beecher, M.D., discovered that much of the pain could be controlled by saline injections. He injected the soldiers with what they thought was morphine, but it was just salt water. Nevertheless, the soldiers felt their pain decrease. Dr. Beecher coined the term "placebo effect," and his subsequent research demonstrated that up to 35 percent of a therapeutic response to any medical treatment could be the result of belief alone.

The placebo effect has been denigrated by some doctors as of little importance. But, I see it as just the opposite. If the placebo is just a prop that allows the mind to control what the body is feeling and doing, then the mind is the medicine. I have always believed in the power of the mind and what it can do. The mind controls our body systems. We do not have to think about making our heart beat, or breathing, or having our billions of cells perform the varied functions that keep us alive. These activities happen by themselves. But many are still controlled and coordinated by parts of our mind. Just because these activities go on without our conscious thought does not mean that they are independent of our control. For example, I believe that the subconscious can affect our body processes for good or bad. I also believe that this type of control is part of what makes us human, but that most of us have forgotten how to use this important ability.

The Subconscious

Perhaps, one reason we have forgotten how to use it is because we live in an age of believing only our five senses. To access the subconscious, however, requires an act of faith. For example, to have your subconscious mind accept directions and control from your conscious mind you have to believe in the idea you are giving your subconscious 100%. You also need to be clear and consistent. For example, I use the image of a CAT scan of my cancer – the white areas that light up on the film, and see my T cells moving to these white areas and killing the cancer. I believe in this 100%. There is no doubt in my mind at all. Why should there be? It is my body. No other person is in control of its processes except me.

If you don't believe there is a connection between the subconscious, the conscious, and the way our bodies work you can try a simple experiment. Read a book like "How You Can Bowl Better Using Self Hypnosis." Bowl a few games before and after you read the book and compare your results. My average score was 170. After I read the book I started bowling many games in the high 200's with a more relaxed stroke and confidence. Obviously bowling is not cancer, but evidence from multiple studies with various types of cancer patients suggests that mind-body interventions can improve mood, quality of life, and coping, as well as lessen disease and treatment-related symptoms, such as chemotherapy-induced nausea, vomiting, and pain.

If the mind can help a patient address how they react to a disease and pain, can it do more? Can the mind actually help heal? Some studies have suggested that mind-body interventions can alter various immune parameters. If the immune system can help manage cancer, then there is hard-wired biological connection between the mind and the control of this disease.

Mind-Body and Immunity

There is considerable evidence that emotional traits, both negative and positive, influence people's susceptibility to infection. For example, following systematic exposure to a respiratory virus in the laboratory, individuals who report higher levels of stress or negative moods have been shown to develop more severe illness than those who report less stress or more positive moods.

69

I think this is true. I know from my own experience that when I feel angry and stressed out long enough I am more likely to get sick.

Psychoneuroimmunology

Psychoneuroimmunology (PNI) takes a scientific approach to this connection between the mind and the immune system. Technically it is defined as the study of the interaction between psychological processes and the nervous and immune systems of the human body. The field of PNI is new and interdisciplinary and connects the fields of psychology, neuroscience, immunology, physiology, pharmacology, psychiatry, behavioral medicine, infectious diseases, endocrinology, rheumatology and others.

What is fascinating about PNI is that the evidence of a mind-body connection is now being discovered. Remember, that such a connection supposedly did not exist and this led to the separation of the mind from the body during the Enlightenment era. For example, in 1981 Dr. David Felten, then working at the Indiana University of Medicine, discovered a network of nerves leading to blood vessels as well as cells of the immune system. The researchers also found nerves in the thymus and spleen terminating near clusters of lymphocytes, macrophages and mast cells, all of which help control immune function. And in 1985, research by neuropharmacologist, Candace Pert, revealed that neuropeptides are present on both the cell walls of the brain and in the immune system. These discoveries suggest that emotions, mental state, and health are deeply interdependent. In fact, they provide the biological mechanisms that explain how neuro-immune interaction occurs and that nerves and neuropeptides wire the brain to the immune system.

Let's think about this. The immune system is a complex surveillance system that is always on patrol throughout the body. The immune cells, called lymphocytes (white blood cells) are the keys to the immune system. One type of cell is the natural killer (NK) cell that attacks and destroys cells that are mutated or

70

abnormal. It is this action which possibly prevents most people from getting cancer.

Now, research has indicated that a link exists between our emotions, which includes all the stress in our lives, and the regulatory systems of the endocrine and immune systems through the central nervous system. This means that our immune system has cells designed to attack cancer cells, but that our state of mind may control how efficiently that system works.

The hard science that proves the mind-body connection is still in its infancy because it had been ignored up until recently. Nonetheless, research is beginning to demonstrate what many of us already know – how we feel and think influences our state of health.

Methods of Mind-Body Medicine

Mind-body medicine typically focuses on strategies that are thought to promote health through relaxation, hypnosis, guided imagery or visualization and biofeedback.

Relaxation

Stress really is a killer. It has been known for a long time that stress can bring about heart attacks and other cardiovascular problems. But stress also can cause or contribute to many other diseases too.

For example, according to researchers at the Institute for Behavioral Medicine Research at Ohio State University, psychological stress disrupts the interaction between the nervous and immune systems which can reduce immune response, slow wound healing, reactivate latent viruses, and enhance the risk for more severe infectious disease.[41]

---

[41] Godbout JP and Glaser R. Stress-induced immune dysregulation: implications for wound healing, infectious disease and cancer. J Neuroimmune Pharmacol. 2006 Dec;1(4):421-7.

Based on what I have learned and the people I have spoken to, some 90% of cancer patients had some stressful time in the previous year and a half prior to diagnosis. And I have noted that many people who have a cancer recurrence have had a stressful period within the previous eight or nine months. Is this just a coincidence?

I know that for me, my stress and the status of my mesothelioma are deeply intertwined. For example, I have measured my stress level every day for three month periods. This is a subjective assessment of how I feel. Then using, CT's, MRI's, tumor markers or my own physical sense of my condition such as pain, I measure the status of my cancer. For me, these two measurements always move up and down together.

Stress Reduction

Stress is much like faith. It is a driving force in our lives. It can be defined, yet never seen. One can only see the results. The first part of reducing stress is recognizing when it attacks and when it is affecting your life. The next step is to back track to find the cause which might be from family, financial worries, or the fears of consequences of the disease. Sometimes stress can come from an event in the past. One of the first things my hypnotherapist and I did was attempt to go back as far as I could remember and resolve any and all conflicts in my past. This is an ongoing process as sometimes things will pop up which I will suddenly recall. But, regardless of the source of the stress, when it hits I can hear "Mr Meso" saying, "Hi there, don't forget about me!" Stress can reactivate cancer.

Self Hypnosis

Because stress can drive or at least encourage cancer, I take steps to reduce it wherever possible. Self hypnosis as been one tool I have used. For example, I relax and think about a quiet and peaceful valley filled with trees and plants and a little stream running through with benches to sit. I imagine sitting there with good friends and relatives (both dead and alive) seeking their wisdom and counsel. Reliving past events and working them out to some type of conclusion. I also use this special place as a source of regeneration where I can lie down and let life flow through creating a happy relaxing atmosphere.

In this valley I also have a "cave" in one of the hillsides. The only way to enter the cave is through a large heavy metal door; the kind that secure giant bank safes. If there is a conflict causing more stress than I can resolve, I open this great door, throw the conflicts into the cave and slam the door shut. In this manner I can rid myself of conflicts, but possibly come back in the future to open the door and resolve it if I choose. This example is a form of "visualization" or "guided imagery."

Physical

Exercise is another wonderful way to relieve stress. Sometimes I will go down to the driving range and hit a bucket of golf balls. Other times I will get on one of the exercise machines, swim laps in the pool at our exercise facility, or just take a walk. Sports are great too. I will play tennis, golf, table tennis, or bowl. Any kind of regular exercise can reduce one's level of stress.

Biofeedback

The word "biofeedback" was coined in the late 1960s to describe the altering of brain activity, blood pressure, heart rate, and other bodily functions that are not normally controlled voluntarily. The most common forms of biofeedback today are the electromyographic (EMG) and the electrodermal (EDR). These sensors allow the person to monitor their own muscle relaxation, heart rate, breathing patterns and perspiration, and concentrate on changing it through either the visual or auditory information provided by the equipment.

Research has demonstrated that biofeedback can help in the treatment of many diseases and conditions. Most patients who benefit from biofeedback are trained to relax and modify their behavior. Most scientists believe that relaxation is a key component in biofeedback treatment.

What Methods Should You Use?

Whatever methods you decide to use, the goals are the same. You want to relax your body and your mind, remove stress, and give yourself positive uplifting and powerful messages of health and life. Think of it as programming your mental computer with the right software so that it performs optimally. The software is the message. You are the computer. Of course, if you do not believe that such programming is possible, you are wasting your time. So the very first step is to decide whether mind-body medicine can really help you. If you believe that it can then you should give it 100% of your belief. You will also need some tools. You can work with a practitioner or with any of the many tapes or books specifically on this subject.

๕ 8 ๛

MAKING TREATMENT
DECISIONS

MAKING A TREATMENT DECISION IS EASY. Making the right one can be very hard. There is no one treatment or healing path that is right for everybody. Some patients reading this book will get a benefit from surgery and chemo. Others will get very little benefit. Some will get a benefit from other approaches like the ones I have described. Others will get no benefit. So how do you decide?

There are two concepts to consider. One is information. The other is intuition.

Information almost goes without saying. You can't make informed treatment decisions unless you have the best information possible. This means talking to and also asking questions of all doctors who are recommending a certain line of treatment. In the Appendix, I have provided some examples of questions you may want to ask. It is important that you are not a passive listener. You need to ask critical questions and be your own advocate.

But doctors can only discuss their own knowledge and experience with you and some doctors are knowledgeable and experienced in some approaches and ignorant of others. For example, asking a conventional medical oncologist about dietary changes is like asking an auto mechanic for a recommendation on a dishwasher. It's not their area of expertise. If you want to learn about diet discuss these questions with a medical doctor trained in this area or a naturopathic doctor or nutritionist or another professional clinician who has actually studied this extensively.

In addition, you may want to learn about all your treatment options – conventional, clinical trials and alternative or complementary. The National Cancer Institute has a database of the various clinical trials currently recruiting patients. The web address is: http://www.cancer.gov/search/clinical_trials

Once you have examined all the appropriate options you are still faced with the decision – what do I choose? This is where intuition comes in. I am not suggesting that you make an emotional decision. That is not what I mean by intuition. Rather, I mean listen to what your gut tells you. Some of us are more in tune to listening to our intuition than others, but listening to inner feelings can be important. There are probably millions of examples of people who made better decisions of all kinds because they listened to their intuition or gut.

How you weigh intuition versus information is a very personal matter. Some of us, especially men are very right brain oriented and will probably listen to our intuition very little. Women are much better at tapping into this other side. All I am suggesting is that after you collect the best data and information possible about your treatment decisions that you allow your intuition to express an opinion too.

Finally, my wish to all those who are reading my book is that you remember that there are long term survivors of this disease. What do we long-term survivors have in common? Most of us took control of our health. You can too and therefore you have a reason to be optimistic. Use the tools and resources available to you to make the best treatments decisions you can. It is your body, your life, and your decisions. No one else's. It is up to you. You can do it!

ᔕ Appendix One ᘔ

DIETARY REFERENCES

The following tables contain data from Dietary Reference Intakes that are published by the National Academy of Sciences. According to the National Academy of Sciences, "Recommended Daily Allowances (RDA) are set to meet the needs of almost all (97-98% of individuals in a group." However, it is unclear if these RDA's apply to people with chronic diseases like cancer. Also, according to the National Academy of Sciences, "Adequate Intakes (AI) is believed to cover the needs of all individuals in the group, but lack of data or uncertainty in the data prevent being able to specify with confidence the percentage of individuals covered by this intake." Again, it is unclear if these numbers are designed to include people with cancer.

As you have read, I often take a lot more of these vitamins and elements than what our country's prestigious scientific establishment recommends. However, as I have stated many times, I do this under the care of trained clinicians. If you wish to exceed the recommendations set forth by the National Academy of Sciences only do it if you are being treated by a licensed clinician. <u>Don't do it on your own</u>!

In the tables that follow, the units of measure are:

- ug/day = microgram/day
- mg/day = milligram/day
- g/day = gram/day

Disclaimer and Warning!

A reasonable attempt was made to report these Dietary Reference Intakes accurately. However, since these reference intakes may change and we cannot guarantee the accuracy of the information appearing in the tables we created, we strongly recommend that you visit the U.S. Department of Agriculture's website for the most accurate, comprehensive, and up-to-date Dietary Reference Intakes available.

Vitamin	Vitamin A	Vitamin C	Vitamin D	Vitamin E	Vitamin K
Unit of Measure and Frequency	ug/day	mg/day	ug/day	mg/day	ug/day
RDA or AI	RDA	RDA	AI	RDA	AI
Note	a		b, c	d	
Males					
9-13	600	45	5	11	60
14-18	900	75	5	15	75
19-30	900	90	5	15	120
31-50	900	90	5	15	120
51-70	900	90	10	15	120
>70	900	90	15	15	120
Females					
9-13	600	45	5	11	60
14-18	700	65	5	15	75
19-30	700	75	5	15	90
31-50	700	75	5	15	90
51-70	700	75	10	15	90
>70	700	75	15	15	90

Vitamin	Thiamin	Riboflavin	Niacin	Vitamin B6	Folate
Unit of Measure and Frequency	mg/day	mg/day	mg/day	mg/day	ug/day
RDA or AI	RDA	RDA	RDA	RDA	RDA
Note			e		f, i
Males					
9-13	0.9	0.9	12	1	300
14-18	1.2	1.3	16	1.3	400
19-30	1.2	1.3	16	1.3	400
31-50	1.2	1.3	16	1.3	400
51-70	1.2	1.3	16	1.7	400
>70	1.2	1.3	16	1.7	400
Females					
9-13	0.9	0.9	12	1	300
14-18	1.0	1.0	14	1.2	400
19-30	1.1	1.1	14	1.3	400
31-50	1.1	1.1	14	1.3	400
51-70	1.1	1.1	14	1.5	400
>70	1.1	1.1	14	1.5	400

Vitamin	Vitamin B12	Pantothenic Acid	Biotin	Choline
Unit of Measure and Frequency	ug/day	mg/day	ug/day	mg/day
RDA or AI	RDA	AI	AI	AI
Note	h, i			g
Males				
9-13	1.8	4	20	375
14-18	2.4	5	25	550
19-30	2.4	5	30	550
31-50	2.4	5	30	550
51-70	2.4	5	30	550
>70	2.4	5	30	550
Females				
9-13	1.8	4	20	375
14-18	2.4	5	25	400
19-30	2.4	5	30	425
31-50	2.4	5	30	425
51-70	2.4	5	30	425
>70	2.4	5	30	425

Elements	Calcium	Chromium	Copper	Fluoride	Iodine
Unit of Measure and Frequency	mg/day	ug/day	ug/day	mg/day	ug/day
RDA or AI	AI	AI	RDA	AI	RDA
Note					
Males					
9-13	1300	25	700	2	120
14-18	1300	35	890	3	150
19-30	1000	35	900	4	150
31-50	1000	35	900	4	150
51-70	1200	30	900	4	150
>70	1200	30	900	4	150
Females					
9-13	1300	21	700	2	120
14-18	1300	24	890	3	150
19-30	1000	25	900	3	150
31-50	1000	25	900	3	150
51-70	1200	20	900	3	150
>70	1200	20	900	3	150

Elements	Iron	Magnesium	Manganese	Molybdenum	Phosphorus
Unit of Measure and Frequency	mg/day	mg/day	mg/day	ug/day	mg/day
RDA or AI	RDA	RDA	AI	RDA	RDA
Note					
Males					
-13	8	240	1.9	34	1250
4-18	11	410	2.2	43	1250
9-30	8	400	2.3	45	700
1-50	8	420	2.3	45	700
1-70	8	420	2.3	45	700
70	8	420	2.3	45	700
Females					
-13	8	240	1.6	34	1250
4-18	15	360	1.6	43	1250
9-30	18	310	1.8	45	700
1-50	18	320	1.8	45	700
1-70	8	320	1.8	45	700
70	8	320	1.8	45	700

Elements	Selenium	Zinc	Potassium	Sodium	Chloride
Unit of Measure and Frequency	ug/day	mg/day	g/day	g/day	g/day
RDA or AI	RDA	RDA	AI	AI	AI
Note					
Males					
9-13	40	8	4.5	1.5	2.3
14-18	55	11	4.7	1.5	2.3
19-30	55	11	4.7	1.5	2.3
31-50	55	11	4.7	1.5	2.3
51-70	55	11	4.7	1.3	2.0
>70	55	11	4.7	1.2	1.8
Females					
9-13	40	8	4.5	1.5	2.3
14-18	55	9	4.7	1.5	2.3
19-30	55	8	4.7	1.5	2.3
31-50	55	8	4.7	1.5	2.3
51-70	55	8	4.7	1.3	2.0
>70	55	8	4.7	1.2	1.8

Notes

These notes are taken verbatim from the Dietary Reference Intakes tables that are published by the National Academy of Sciences.

a) As retinol activity equivalents (RAEs). 1 RAE = 1 mg retinol, 12 mg b-carotene, 24 mg a-carotene, or 24 mg b-cryptoxanthin. The RAE for dietary provitamin A carotenoids is twofold greater than retinol equivalents (RE), whereas the RAE for preformed vitamin A is the same as RE.

b) As cholecalciferol. 1 µg cholecalciferol = 40 IU vitamin D.

c) In the absence of adequate exposure to sunlight.

d) As a-tocopherol. a-Tocopherol includes RRR-a-tocopherol, the only form of a-tocopherol that occurs naturally in foods, and the 2R-stereoisomeric forms of a-tocopherol (RRR-, RSR-, RRS-, and RSS-a-tocopherol) that occur in fortified foods and supplements. It does not include the 2S-stereoisomeric forms of a-tocopherol (SRR-, SSR-, SRS-, and SSS-a-tocopherol), also found in fortified foods and supplements.

e) As niacin equivalents (NE). 1 mg of niacin = 60 mg of tryptophan; 0–6 months = preformed niacin (not NE).

f) As dietary folate equivalents (DFE). 1 DFE = 1 µg food folate = 0.6 µg of folic acid from fortified food or as a supplement consumed with food = 0.5 µg of a supplement taken on an empty stomach.

g) Although AIs have been set for choline, there are few data to assess whether a dietary supply of choline is needed at all stages of the life cycle, and it may be that the choline requirement can be met by endogenous synthesis at some of these stages.

h) Because 10 to 30 percent of older people may malabsorb food-bound B12, it is advisable for those older than 50 years to meet their RDA mainly by consuming foods fortified with B12 or a supplement containing B12.

i) In view of evidence linking folate intake with neural tube defects in the fetus, it is recommended that all women capable of becoming pregnant consume 400 µg from supplements or fortified foods in addition to intake of food folate from a varied diet.

j) It is assumed that women will continue consuming 400 µg from supplements or fortified food until their pregnancy is confirmed and they enter prenatal care, which ordinarily occurs after the end of the periconceptional period—the critical time for formation of the neural tube.

ℬ Appendix Two ℭ

QUESTIONS TO ASK YOUR DOCTORS

HERE ARE EIGHT QUESTIONS TO CONSIDER WHEN YOU ARE DISCUSSING CANCER TREATMENT OPTIONS WITH YOUR DOCTORS.

1. Is it alright if I tape this conversation?

When life and death decisions are at stake, conversations with oncologists and other physicians take on enormous importance. In addition, sometimes these conversations take place when the doctor is very busy. Given the subject, the hurried bedside manner of some physicians, and the emotional intensity for the patient and family, it can be very hard to listen, understand, and ask appropriate questions. Tape recording important conversations with your doctor(s) about treatment options is an excellent way to provide a record so that you can: 1) concentrate on listening; 2) do not have to worry about taking notes; 3) can focus on your questions; 4) can replay and review the conversation in a less stressful environment such as your own home to fully comprehend what the physician communicated.

An added benefit is that recording the conversation can facilitate more time with the doctor. When the oncologist knows the conversation is taped they may actually give you a few extra minutes. Furthermore, it provides an advantage to both you and your doctors if there is ever a question later about what was or was not promised.

Do not secretly tape record anyone. In many jurisdictions this is against the law. You should always obtain permission by telling your doctor(s) that you want a tape recording of the meeting/consultation so that you can review it later or you wish to share the conversation with a family member who could not be present at the meeting. In fact, it is always a good idea to use the first few seconds of the recording to have all the parties acknowledge that the meeting is being recorded with their permission.

2. Did you send my pathology (report and slides) to another hospital for a second opinion?

The pathology of your tumor cells tells pathologists whether you actually have cancer and what kind. Having a second look/opinion by another pathologist from another hospital helps ensure that you have been properly diagnosed. There have been unfortunate situations when patients have been treated inappropriately because the wrong kind of cancer was diagnosed. In many hospitals it is standard practice to "send the slides out" for a second opinion. You may want to check to ensure this step was taken in your case and find out who rendered the second opinion and what they concluded.

3. Do you have any financial or research interest in this treatment you are recommending? For example, are you being paid by a drug company when you prescribe these drugs? Do you consult for the drug company that makes these drugs?

Some oncologists have financial arrangements with various drug makers or other financial incentives that could be construed as a conflict of interest. You should find out whether your doctor(s) has any financial or research interest in recommending a certain treatment.

4. **How many patients have you treated with my exact same cancer? Same age and same cancer? Which treatments did you use? Are any of the patients still alive? Can I speak with them?**

You want to get a good idea of what the oncologist's experience is with the various treatments being recommended. You should find out how many patients (your age with the exact same cancer) they have treated with each therapy. Ask if you can speak to these other patients. Other patients (like you) who have been administered the same therapy by the same oncologist(s) can provide valuable insight into what to expect.

5. **Did any patients have side-effects from the treatment? What were they? What was the worse side-effect? Did anyone die from the treatment, not the cancer?**

Some patients do not die from their cancer, but die from the treatment. You should ask questions to learn how toxic the therapy is.

6. **Are these drugs FDA approved for treating my cancer?**

Many cancer drugs are not FDA-approved for the use for which they are prescribed. (This is called "off-label" use.) In fact, some drugs that are widely used for a particular cancer may never have been approved for safety or efficacy for that use by the FDA. It is valuable to know if any of the drugs the oncologist intends to prescribe would be used "off label" and if so, why the oncologist is comfortable with that use.

7. Can you show me where the survival information comes from? Is it reported in the peer-reviewed published medical literature? Can you give me a copy of the article?

Cancer Monthly www.cancermonthly.com provides survival information from the medical/scientific literature - journals your doctors should be familiar with. The oncologist should be able to support any survival/prognosis claim they may make with data or published studies that they can share with you. Be wary, if they can not support their claims of a potential cure with medical studies or with examples of other patients they have treated.

8. What is my prognosis with no treatment?

Comparisons are very seldom made between the results of a clinical trial and those patients who received no adjuvant treatment (i.e. no therapy beyond surgery). When survival and quality of life comparisons are made, they are usually made between two or more treatments, not between treatment and no treatment. It is very difficult, therefore, for an oncologist to objectively answer the question how long did the treated patients live and what was their quality of life compared to those who received no adjuvant therapy. Nonetheless, it may be of interest to ask your doctor for a reference/study that discusses this. Be advised that such studies may not be available.

∽ Appendix Three ∾

INTERVIEW WITH PAUL KRAUS

PAUL KRAUS IS A FELLOW MESOTHELIOMA SURVIVOR WHO CONTINUES TO DO WELL ELEVEN YEARS AFTER BEGING TOLD THAT HE HAD LESS THAN A YEAR TO LIVE. He has followed many of the same regimens I have. Like me he has never had any conventional therapy (chemotherapy, radiation, or surgery) and has used a variety of natural approaches. Below is an interview he gave to Cancer Monthly back in 2005. More information about him can be found on his website: www.survivingmesothelioma.com

Surviving Mesothelioma, a Terminal Cancer:
Paul Kraus' Remarkable Story

For anyone faced with a dire prognosis of cancer or any other disease, the following interview will inspire you. In the annals of cancer, mesothelioma is one of the worst possible types of cancer to have. In the words of oncologists it has a "dismal therapeutic outcome" and is "an aggressive incurable tumor." The median survival from diagnosis ranges from 6 to 18 months. Despite this prognosis, Mr. Paul Kraus is alive ten years after he was diagnosed with peritoneal mesothelioma. What is equally remarkable is that Mr. Kraus had no orthodox cancer therapies -

he opted to say 'no' to chemotherapy, surgery, and radiation. Instead, Mr. Kraus made radical lifestyle changes, altering his diet, using intravenous and oral vitamins, herbs, amino acids and other immune boosting therapies and supplements, and tapping into the power of the mind-body connection.

The Diagnosis

Cancer Monthly: Paul can you tell us when you were diagnosed and what types of symptoms you experienced that led to your diagnosis?

PK: I was diagnosed at the end of June 1997. The only symptom I had was a very bloated abdomen. I did not have any pain. I actually went into the hospital for an umbilical hernia repair and the cancer was an accidental finding. During the surgery the surgeon removed a lot of fluid from my abdomen. He also conducted a laparoscopic examination that revealed widespread metastases. He first thought that I had metastatic pancreatic cancer. It took two or three weeks for the pathology to come back from Sydney and say that in fact it was mesothelioma.

Cancer Monthly: And that diagnosis was reconfirmed by another hospital?

PK: Yes, my pathology was sent to Australia's leading pathologist in mesothelioma cases, Professor Douglas Henderson of Adelaide. They had two teams of pathologists verify and confirm the diagnosis. In fact, it was confirmed as peritoneal or abdominal rather than pleural mesothelioma. This is a very unusual subtype, even within the annals of mesothelioma.

Cancer Monthly: Does peritoneal mesothelioma have the same kind of dire prognosis as the more frequently encountered pleural mesothelioma?

PK: Yes. In fact, when we first went to a professor of oncology in Sydney, we thought that peritoneal is less dangerous than pleural. He shook his head and said, "Oh, no, oh no. In fact, in some ways it is even more difficult."

Cancer Monthly: How was your health history prior to that diagnosis?

PK: It had been good, but I had suffered from a lot of stress. And there were minor family traumas in the previous 12 to 18 months before diagnosis. Some writers say that things like that may affect one's immune function. Sometimes I conjecture whether that was a little warning or a tap on the shoulder from someone upstairs to change my lifestyle, which I of course I radically did, but more about that in a few minutes.

Previous Exposure to Asbestos

Cancer Monthly: Now, mesothelioma regardless of the subtype is associated with prior exposure to asbestos. Had you been exposed to asbestos?

PK: For the first 12 or 18 months after my diagnosis I did not make the connection that about 35 years earlier I had been exposed to asbestos. I am a former high school teacher. I did not work with asbestos in any way. But, in the early 1960's when I was a university student and on my vacation, I was working in a factory where they were sawing asbestos fiber sheets nearby. There, I was exposed to that blue dust for a few weeks. Nobody warned me. There were no warnings, no signs. This was the only known source of exposure for me. After leaving university I became a high school teacher and a writer. So I had no other known exposure. In fact, my early medical records stated that this patient has no known exposure to asbestos. The disease lay dormant for all that time.

Cancer Monthly: Did you file suit?

93

PK: I did eventually take up proceedings (sue). I was very very reluctant to do this. In fact I flatly refused. However, I was prompted by my son. He pointed out correctly what this diagnosis has done to my life. How my income had been slashed, and so on. I finally succumbed to these promptings and succeeded in gaining compensation for my damages.

Treatment Choices

Cancer Monthly: Now, you are faced with this horrible diagnosis and I imagine you are being offered perhaps surgery, chemotherapy or radiation. Instead you opted not to have any orthodox treatments. Can you tell us how you came to make these decisions?

PK: Actually, I was not offered much hope at all. My medical prognosis was very poor. At that time, I asked what were the chances of success with chemotherapy and I was told not very high at all. That's why I opted for a different path. Apart from being racked with fear and the fact that the fluid in my abdomen was building up again, I did not have any pain. My quality of life was, at that moment, okay. I made the decision not to go down that so called conventional path because I was told by the doctors that my quality of life would be quite severely compromised with the heavy chemotherapy I would have been prescribed. And so I made a major decision. I decided to radically change my lifestyle. I read books by Bernie Siegel (Peace, Love and Healing: Bodymind Communication & the Path to Self-Healing: An Exploration; Love, Medicine and Miracles: Lessons Learned about Self-Healing from a Surgeon's Experience with Exceptional Patients). I read books by Andrew Weil (Spontaneous Healing), and Simonton and Matthews (Getting Well Again). These books were incredibly inspirational and useful. For example, Andrew Weil wrote that any illness can be conquered through radical lifestyle change because our bodies are made with powerful self-healing capacities. It was damn hard

94

to make such radical changes, but I was determined to see them through. I realized that to do otherwise meant that my chances of surviving were greatly diminished.

I made the decision that I am going to do everything I possibly can to turn this illness around. I began juicing --- carrot juice and beetroot juice, as well as green juices four or five times a day. I learned to meditate and use visualization. I did this for hours. I also prayed. I went to prayer groups and healing groups. I learned affirmations. I radically altered my diet into a vegetarian diet. I cut-out sugar. I ate high-fiber, predominantly raw food, but not exclusively. I also focused on exercise. I began taking vitamin, mineral, herbal and homeopathic supplements along with amino acids (N-Acetyl-Cystine (NAC), methylcobalamin, reduced glutathione). Also I took vitamins A, C, and E. Non-acidic vitamin C. Calcium ascorbate powder. I take slightly less now than I what I did initially. For the first couple of years after the diagnosis I was taking 8 grams a day in divided doses of Vitamin C in the form of calcium ascorbate.

Cancer Monthly: Were you taking the Vitamin C orally or intravenously.

PK: I took the 8 grams orally, it's in powder form and I dissolved it in water. But one of the therapies that I count as very important in those early days was the intravenous vitamin C that I had administered in conjunction with what is called ozone therapy.

Cancer Monthly: And how was the ozone therapy administered?

PK: Intravenously. They took blood out of a vein, used an ozone machine to ozone the blood and reintroduced it into my body through a drip. The rationale for that was that cancer does not like an oxygenated environment and the ozone therapy greatly helped to oxygenate the cells. In addition, I used another treatment when I was first diagnosed called Ukrain. These treatments were an adjunct to my lifestyle change.

The other thing I should say that I think is terribly important, almost fundamental, is that for the first four or five months after diagnosis, the volume of fluid in my abdomen was not really improving. I complained to my doctor, I said, "Look I'm doing all this and nothing is happening." And he reminded me, admonished me actually, and he said, "Be patient because this takes time. You are getting better. You affirm that you are getting better in your affirmations and your visualizations which you use in conjunction with these therapies. So just give it time." And he was right. His words were prophetic. They did in fact stabilize my cancer.

Cancer Monthly: For the treatments you mentioned, the Ukrain, ozone therapy, Vitamin C, supplements, other vitamins, how were you able to put that regimen or protocol together? Did you find it all in one place or in parts from your research and reading?

PK: This protocol or regime came about from my intensive research. I did not have access to the internet at that stage, back in 1997, but a friend did. We researched it together. Also, I had by great fortune a holistic doctor, a general practitioner. He routinely used intravenous C for other cancer patients. That particular aspect of the protocol was through him. He also said he had heard about Ukrain but that he did not know very much about it. So we tracked it down and incorporated it into my treatment and the same with the ozone therapy. He had said that he did not know too much about ozone therapy but that in my situation it was worth a try.

Cancer Monthly: That's absolutely fantastic that you had an open-minded holistic practitioner who was willing to try things with you.

PK: Yes.

Cancer Monthly: In terms of the timeline, did you start this protocol soon after your diagnosis or was there a period where you waited? How quickly did you start all of this?

PK: The radical lifestyle change especially regarding diet, I started virtually immediately. The juicing and changing of my diet to the vegetarian, low fat, no sugar I started literally within a few days of being diagnosed. Now for the supplements, within a month I was on the basic vitamins A, C, and E. Then gradually over the first few months after that I learned about some of these minerals such as selenium which is a very important and the amino acids and so on. I started on intravenous C within 6 weeks of diagnosis. And I learned to meditate. I was reading the books that I mentioned earlier within a couple of weeks after I was diagnosed.

Cancer Monthly: How are you doing now?

PK: Four months ago I turned sixty and I feel fine. I live day to day. My tests are okay. They say that I still have cancer and my energy level is not very good. But, I'm fine. I don't have any pain. My doctor tells me, "You're fine. Just keep up what you are doing and you will go on for years." He's convinced of it because the CT scans do not show any deterioration. They do vary a bit. They do show there is still fluid, but I have affirmed that sure there's fluid in there but it's probably non-malignant by now.

Cancer Monthly: And from the time of your diagnosis until now you have never had chemotherapy, radiation, or surgery?

PK: That is correct. In fact in August 2000, I was under a great deal of stress because one of my children was very ill. My condition began to deteriorate and I saw an eminent cancer surgeon. He recommended that I have a very major surgery. What is called a peritonectomy where they remove, over 10 or

12 hours, the entire peritoneal lining. And I really meditated on that, I thought about it. I asked my general practitioner about it. He said, "Look even though the test shows a deterioration, how are you feeling?" I said, "I feel fine. I don't have any pain." He said, "Go back on the intravenous C. Go back on the Ukrain. Go back on the ozone therapy." And he felt confident that since I had done it once before I could do it again. And he was right. So I did not have surgery.

Cancer Monthly: So you went back on the protocol in August 2000 and stayed on it for how long?

PK: About 14 or 15 months. I know if this happens again I'll just return to that full IV protocol.

Cancer Monthly: And now you are doing what one might call maintenance therapy?

PK: That's exactly right.

Cancer Monthly: And that's comprised of the oral vitamins, minerals, other supplements, and diet?

PK: That is correct.

Cancer Monthly: You have talked about the importance of the regimen and also the importance of a positive mental state. Would you say that your mental state is as essential as the therapies?

PK: Absolutely. I would be giving a false impression if I were to say I was psychologically on top of things from the beginning. I was not, especially in the first six months after diagnosis. At that point, it was not so much a struggle against cancer as it was a struggle with myself, with my constant fears and doubts. That was my battle. I was battling myself as much as I was the cancer. There is something terribly important here. As part of my therapy, I wrote a journal which ultimately became a book called Faith, Hope, Love and Laugher: How They Heal. It was highly therapeutic in my case just writing down thoughts and fears and doubts; chronicling these sorts of things.

Also, I'll never forget the first day that I had those intravenous therapies administered. I was very fearful. The nurse who was doing the administrating detected my fears. She put everything down and said, "I want you to affirm, visualize as I administer these therapies that they are actually doing you good. This is very important and powerful to your healing. If you don't accept that these therapies are doing you good then the treatment will not work because your mind and your body are one." She was right. The mind body connection is very important for healing. They are inextricably linked. If one has the wrong attitude one cannot be a survivor of mesothelioma or any form of cancer.

১০ Appendix Four ৫৪

PATHOLOGY DIAGNOSIS

THIS ARTICLE IS REPRINTED WITH PERMISSION FROM CANCERWIRE. It discusses the importance of considering a second pathology opinion. I thought it would be appropriate to reprint because mesothelioma can be a difficult cancer to diagnose correctly.

Pathology Diagnosis: Do You Need a Second Opinion?

John, age eight, was diagnosed with an Anaplastic Astrocytoma (AA) which is an aggressive and often fatal brain tumor. He underwent brain surgery followed by high-dose chemotherapy and radiation therapy (equivalent to about 50,000 dental x-rays). These treatments are highly toxic to the developing brain of a child and, if he were to survive, his IQ and cognitive abilities would be seriously compromised. The family moved to a different state and took John to the local children's hospital for follow-up care. There, the doctors reviewed John's pathology slides. They discovered that John's tumor was not an AA, but was benign. This diagnosis was subsequently confirmed by two other hospitals. John never needed chemotherapy or radiation therapy. Today, John's IQ decreases at a rate of about 6 points a year as he suffers from the side-effects of a treatment he never needed.

Pathology is the medical specialty that deals with the examination of tissues and cells under the microscope in order to arrive at a diagnosis. When it comes to cancer, a pathological diagnosis is the gold standard that indicates the presence or absence of cancer, the type of cancer, and its classification. Because therapeutic decisions are based on the presumed reliability of the pathology diagnosis, a misdiagnosis can result in unnecessary, harmful and aggressive therapy (like John's story) or inadequate treatment. Unfortunately, medical studies over the last two decades have demonstrated that this gold standard is not consistently reliable. In fact, multiple studies have demonstrated discrepancy rates of up to 30% with an average of approximately 10%. A "discrepancy" happens when one pathologist renders a diagnosis and another pathologist looks at the same material and renders a different opinion. See for example, Gupta D and Layfield LJ, Prevalence of inter-institutional anatomic pathology slide review: a survey of current practice. Am J Surg Pathol. 2000 Feb;24(2):280-4.

Here are some examples from the medical literature:

Bladder Cancer – Wrong Pathology Would Have Led to Five Unnecessary Cystectomies

The pathology of 97 patients (131 specimens) with suspected urothelial carcinoma of the bladder was reviewed. Twenty-four of the 131 specimens "exhibited significant discrepancies." This included two patients who showed no evidence of tumor. As a result of the review, five radical cystectomies were avoided.

- Coblentz TR, Mills SE, Theodorescu D. Cancer. 2001 Apr 1;91(7):1284-90. Impact of second opinion pathology in the definitive management of patients with bladder carcinoma.

Brain Tumors – Pathologists Often Disagree With Themselves or Others

Pathologists agreed with their original diagnosis only 51.43% for anaplastic astrocytomas, 74.73% for glioblastoma multiforme, and 65.22% for low-grade astrocytomas. Pathologists agreed with other pathologists only 62.41% for glioblastomas, 36.04% for AA, and 57.14% for low-grade astrocytomas.

- Mittler MA, et al., J Neurosurg. 1996 Dec;85(6):1091-4. Observer reliability in histological grading of astrocytoma stereotactic biopsies.

Breast Cancer – Different Treatment Recommendations 43% of the Time

Seventy-five women with a total of 77 breast lesions were examined. The reviewing panel disagreed with the treatment recommendations 43% of the time (32 cases). The disagreements included breast-conservation therapy instead of mastectomy (13 patients) and different treatment based on a "major change in diagnosis on pathology review. (3.9%)."

- Chang JH, et al., Cancer. 2001 Apr 1;91(7):1231-7. The impact of a multidisciplinary breast cancer center on recommendations for patient management: the University of Pennsylvania experience.

Ovarian Cancer – 12.7% Did Not Have Ovarian Cancer

The medical records and pathology slides of 339 women diagnosed with ovarian cancer were reviewed. Forty-three women (12.7%) were discovered not to have ovarian cancer. (28 had other types of cancer and 15 had benign tumors.)

- McGowan L, Norris HJ. Surg Gynecol Obstet. 1991 Sep;173(3):211-5. The mistaken diagnosis of carcinoma of the ovary.

Prostate Cancer – Wrong Pathology Would Have Led to Six Unnecessary Prostatectomies

A total of 535 men referred for radical prostatectomy were reviewed. Seven (1.3%) of the men were found to have a benign pathology. "Upon subsequent clinical work up, six of seven men were considered not to have adenocarcinoma, and their surgery was cancelled."

- Epstein JI, et al., Am J Surg Pathol. 1996 Jul;20(7):851-7. Clinical and cost impact of second-opinion pathology. Review of prostate biopsies prior to radical prostatectomy.

Soft Tissue Lesions – Benign Considered Malignant and Malignant Considered Benign

In this study 266 cases of soft tissue lesions were reviewed. A major discrepancy was found in 25% of cases. Of these discrepancies, 45% consisted of benign lesions diagnosed as sarcomas, and 23% were sarcomas diagnosed as benign tumors.

- Arbiser ZK, Folpe AL, Weiss SW. Am J Clin Pathol. 2001 Oct;116(4):473-6. Consultative (expert) second opinions in soft tissue pathology. Analysis of problem-prone diagnostic situations.

Getting the pathology wrong is not limited to the U.S. Other countries have found similar problems. For example, in the United Kingdom, 413 cases of sarcoma were reviewed and the diagnosis was confirmed only 76% of the time. The study concluded that "second opinion is essential in cases of presumed sarcoma…to ensure that appropriate treatment is selected."

- Harris M, Hartley AL, et al., Br J Cancer. 1991 Aug;64(2):315-20. Sarcomas in north west England: I.Histopathological peer review

Do You Need a Second Opinion?

The vast majority of pathologists are excellent physicians and that the diagnoses they render are correct. However, a minority of cases benefit from a second opinion. The problem, of course, is accurately identifying which cases should get a second opinion. One factor to consider is how rare your cancer is. If it is rare, chances are that your pathologist has not seen many of your type. However, even if your cancer is more common, you might consider erring on the side of caution and requesting a second opinion.

Writing in the journal Cancer, Joseph D Kronz, M.D. and his colleagues at Johns Hopkins Department of Pathology stated, "Second opinion surgical pathology can result in major therapeutic and prognostic modifications for patients sent to large referral hospitals. Although the overall percentage of affected cases is not large, the consistent rate of discrepant diagnosis uncovered by second opinion surgical pathology may have an enormous human and financial impact. Accordingly, the authors recommend that review of the original histologic material should be undertaken prior to the institution of a major therapeutic endeavor."

- Kronz JD, et al., Cancer 1999 Dec 1;86(11):2426-35. Mandatory second opinion surgical pathology at a large referral hospital

Getting a Second Opinion

The microscopic glass slides, pathology reports, and possibly paraffin (wax) blocks taken from your blood, aspirate, or tumor are archived in the pathology department of the hospital where your surgery or biopsy took place. As the patient, you can request that this material be released for the purpose of obtaining a second opinion from another pathologist. You can do this even if you have already started treatment. (Be sure to find out if there is a charge for this, how much, and whether your insurance will pay.) Large academic medical centers where doctors are trained often have the most experienced pathologists. When requesting a second opinion, ask that it be sent to a prominent medical center that sees many patients like you. Also request that the pathologist who actually does the review has special experience with your type of cancer. For example, for brain cancer you would want a neuro-pathologist to perform the review. Your surgeon or oncologist should help facilitate such a second opinion.

ℰ Appendix Five ℛ

RESEARCHING ALTERNATIVE CANCER THERAPIES

This article is also reprinted with permission from CancerWire. It discusses how to conduct valid research on alternative therapies for cancer; a subject of critical importance.

Obtaining Credible Information About Alternative Cancer Therapies

When it comes to alternative therapies for cancer, the internet is a "mixed bag" filled with exaggerated claims, unreliable anecdotes, and some very credible reports. For the patient who has little time and who needs reliable information now, sorting through this can be a challenge. There is, however, one resource that is arguably better than many others. Medline is the National Library of Medicine's bibliographic database covering the fields of medicine, nursing, dentistry, veterinary medicine, the health care system, and the preclinical sciences. Medline contains over 12 million citations and abstracts (summaries of research articles) from more than 4,800 biomedical journals published in the United States and 70 other countries. Medline is accessible from your computer via PubMed, which was developed by the National Center for Biotechnology Information (NCBI). Simply type www.pubmed.gov in your browser. Through Medline you can see what has been published about alternative cancer therapies by scientists and researchers. For anyone trying to make an informed treatment decision, these studies are worth browsing.

For example, certain herbs have been used throughout history for the treatment of various cancers. Because natural substances are difficult to patent, drug companies will not invest money to research and develop these substances. Nonetheless, you can find a handful of studies for almost any herb, vitamin or other substance you may be looking for. Although these studies are obviously not the final word, they do provide clues about the potential efficacy of these agents in cancer. While most of these studies are pre-clinical (in test-tubes, animal models), some are clinical (in patients). Faced with the hyperbole on the internet and the skepticism of most orthodox doctors, these studies can also be used to facilitate objective discussions with your physician.

There are three suggested steps to accessing this information:

Step 1) Go to Medline www.pubmed.gov

Step 2) Run a search by placing terms like the name of the herb or vitamin and cancer. For example, "red clover and breast cancer" or "vitamin c and prostate cancer" or "carrots and lung cancer." If nothing appears, try the Latin name of the substance.

Step 3) Understand what you are reading. While it is advantageous to read the entire article (often available in your local medical library), abstracts of the article are a good place to begin. And while, there are many considerations in assessing an article's reliability (i.e. journal, authors, conflicts of interest, size of study, etc.) for the purpose of getting started, you can begin by focusing on three key pieces of information:

1. What substance was tested?

You want to know what was actually tested. For example, some studies do not use the entire natural product, but only employ one or more chemical components that are isolated or synthesized. A problem with this approach is that all the components may have a synergistic effect and administering one ingredient may not be a fair test of what the agent can really do in patients.

2. Where was it tested?

There are many ways a test can be performed. For example, preclinical testing can be performed in cancer cell cultures (in vitro) which are cultures of cancer cells taken from a patient. Or, it can be performed in a cell line (a cancer cell culture that has been grown and used for years or decades). Or, it can be performed in animals (with animal cancers or human cancers). Or, the test can be performed clinically by administering the agent to actual cancer patients. Of course, the last one would be the most accurate representation of whether the agent works in people.

3. What was the outcome?

Here, you want to know what happened. Key terms to look for include apoptosis (this means the cancer cells committed cell suicide) anti-proliferation, and growth inhibition.

Some examples can be found below. (Please note that Cancer Monthly does not endorse the use of any of these substances for the treatment of your cancer, but encourages you to perform reliable research in order to make informed treatment decisions with your licensed healthcare provider).

Example 1

What was tested: Pau d'Arco is the inner bark of the Tabebuia avellanedae tree. It has been used for centuries by the Indio tribes of South America to treat a wide range of conditions including pain, arthritis, inflammation of the prostate gland (prostatitis), fever, dysentery, boils and ulcers, and various cancers. In this study, the researchers tested beta-lapachone which is a component of Pau d'arco.

Tested in: Cultured human prostate cells.

Result: Growth inhibition and induction of apoptosis in a dose-dependent manner.

Translation: They used only one component of the herb (beta-lapachone) and they tested in it in prostate cancer cells, not prostate cancer patients. The cancer cell stopped growing. This is evidence that these components work in prostate cancer cells (not necessarily patients).

Reference: Lee JH, et al., Down-regulation of cyclooxygenase-2 and telomerase activity by beta-lapachone in human prostate carcinoma cells. Pharmacol Res. 2005 Jun;51(6):553-60.

Example 2

What was tested: Red clover (Trifolium pretense), a wild plant used as grazing food for cattle and other livestock, has been used medicinally to treat a wide array of conditions. Here they tested Red Clover derived dietary isoflavones containing a mixture of genistein, daidzein, formononetin, and biochanin A.

Tested in: Prostate cancer patients.

Result: Apoptosis in radical prostatectomy specimens from treated patients was significantly higher than control subjects.

Translation: They used a variety of the components from Red Clover and they administered it to real patients. The fact that apoptosis was greater in the treated patients (those who received the herb's components) is an indicator of potential efficacy in actual prostate cancer patients.

Reference: Jarred RA, et al., Induction of apoptosis in low to moderate-grade human prostate carcinoma by red clover-derived dietary isoflavones. Cancer Epidemiol Biomarkers Prev. 2002 Dec;11(12):1689-96.

Example 3

What was tested: Cat's Claw (Uncaria tomentosa) is a tropical vine that grows in South America. This vine gets its name from the small thorns at the base of the leaves, which looks like a cat's claw. It has been used in South-American folk medicine for the treatment of cancer, arthritis, gastritis and epidemic diseases. In this study, extracts were used.

Tested in: Human breast cancer cell line

Result: Antiproliferative effect and a 90% inhibition at a concentration of 100 mg/ml.

Translation: Extracts (not the whole plant) were used in a human breast cancer cell line (not cells taken from a recent patient). There were significant anti-proliferative effects which means that the extracts worked in this cell line.

Reference: Riva L, et al., The antiproliferative effects of Uncaria tomentosa extracts and fractions on the growth of breast cancer cell line. Anticancer Res. 2001 Jul-Aug;21(4A):2457-61.

Example 4

What was tested: Curcumin (also called Tumeric) is a yellow powder ground from the root of a plant (Curcuma longa) of the ginger family, which is found wild in the Himalayas and grown across South Asia. In this study they used the whole herb.

Tested in: Patients with bladder cancer or pre-malignant lesions

Result: Histologic improvement in some patients with the precancerous lesions.

Translation: Whole herb (root) was tested in a variety of patients and there was some efficacy in the patients who had pre-malignant cancer.

Reference: Cheng AL, et al., Phase I clinical trial of curcumin, a chemopreventive agent, in patients with high-risk or pre-malignant lesions. Anticancer Res. 2001 Jul-Aug;21(4B):2895-900.

Example 5

What was tested: Vitamin C plasma levels.

Tested in: Patients with advanced cancer.

Result: Patients with low plasma concentrations of vitamin C have a shorter survival.

Translation: In patients with a variety of different advanced cancers, patients with less Vitamin C in their plasma (i.e. blood) did not live as long as those patients who had more.

Reference: Mayland CR, et al., Vitamin C deficiency in cancer patients. Palliat Med. 2005 Jan;19(1):17-20.

Again, the studies indexed in PubMed are not the last word, but when searching for reliable information on the internet, browsing what is published in medical and scientific journals by using Medline is a good place to begin. We encourage you to take advantage of this comprehensive resource to help make informed treatment decisions with your licensed healthcare provider.

ℰ Appendix Six ℜ

MY ALTERNATIVE LICENSED CLINICIANS

Nutritionist

Judith Todero
Todero Counseling
Riverside, CA
Tel. 951-341-5777

Hypnotherapist

Dr. Don Morris
Morris Institute of Hypnotherapy
7177 Brockton Ave, Suite 331
Riverside, CA 92506
Tel. 951-788-2008

ℬ Appendix Seven ℭ

ARTICLES ON CANCER
AND NUTRITION

Additional articles on cancer and nutrition published by
Cancer Monthly. All available online at:
  www.cancermonthly.com or:
  http://www.cancermonthly.com/iNP/category_view_l.asp?CID=3

Prostate Cancer and Magnolia: Magnolia Tree Extract Offers New
Promise for Treating Prostate Cancer. Published by Cancer Monthly,
April 25, 2008.

Flavopiridol and Rhabdoid Tumors: Plant Extract Targets Deadly
Childhood Cancer. Published by Cancer Monthly, April 21, 2008.

Vegan Diet and Cancer: Very-Low-Fat Vegan Diet May Offer Cancer
Protection. Published by Cancer Monthly, April 21, 2008.

Cancer Clinical Trials and Alternative Treatments: Few Clinical Trials
Focus on Alternative Approaches to Cancer. Published by Cancer
Monthly, March 28, 2008.

Targeting the Immune System to Attack Cancer: Helping the body's
immune system to eliminate cancer cells. Published by Cancer
Monthly, February 12, 2008.

Colon Cancer and Red Yeast Rice: Plant Red Yeast Rice Might Help Slow Colon Cancer Growth. Published by Cancer Monthly, December 17, 2007.

Prostate Cancer and Lycopene: Lycopene Shows Benefit in the Treatment of Prostate Cancer. Published by Cancer Monthly, December 12, 2007.

Cancer Pain & Complementary Therapies: A new study examines the role of acupuncture, massage, mind-body techniques, and dietary supplements in dealing with the pain associated with cancer. Published by Cancer Monthly, November 26, 2007.

Chamomile Targets Cancer Cells: Chamomile selectively kills cancer cells and spares normal cells through a process of programmed cell death, or apoptosis. Published by Cancer Monthly, November 20, 2007.

Vitamin C and Cancer: Is Vitamin C a Viable Treatment for Cancer? Published by Cancer Monthly, October 16, 2007.

Small-Cell Lung Cancer and Green Tea: Green tea data show promise in treating small-cell lung carcinoma: Ingredient brings about cell death by reducing activity of key enzyme. Published by Cancer Monthly, August 1, 2007.

Breast Cancer and Medicinal Herb: Medicinal Herb Appears to Hinder Breast Cancer Cells: Data suggests Ocimum gratissimum may help prevent and treat the disease. Published by Cancer Monthly, July 11, 2007.

Antioxidants and Chemotherapy: The Antioxidant-and-Chemotherapy Combo: "Solid and consistent data" shows significant benefits of antioxidants. Published by Cancer Monthly, May 22, 2007.

Cancer Pain & Complementary Therapies: Stopping Bladder Cancer at the Cellular Level – Naturally: Mushroom extracts induce sharp growth reduction in superficial tumor cells. Published by Cancer Monthly, November 26, 2007.

Bladder Cancer and Mushrooms: Stopping Bladder Cancer at the Cellular Level – Naturally: Mushroom extracts induce sharp growth

115

reduction in superficial tumor cells. Published by Cancer Monthly, May 21, 2007.

ℰℐ

INDEX